The Cleveland Clinic Guide to

PAIN MANAGEMENT

Michael Stanton-Hicks, MD

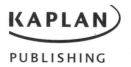

PUBLISHING

New York

This publication is designed to provide accurate and authoritative information in regard to the subject matter covered. It is sold with the understanding that the publisher is not engaged in rendering medical, legal, or other professional service. If medical advice or other expert assistance is required, the services of a competent professional should be sought.

Artwork is reprinted with the permission of the Cleveland Clinic Center for Medical Art & Photography © 2010.

Published by Kaplan Publishing, a division of Kaplan, Inc.
1 Liberty Plaza, 24th Floor
New York, NY 10006

Printed in the United States of America

10 9 8 7 6 5 4 3 2 1

Library of Congress Cataloging-in-Publication Data

Stanton-Hicks, Michael d'A.
    The Cleveland Clinic guide to pain management / Michael Stanton-Hicks.
        p. cm. — (Cleveland Clinic guide series)
    Includes index.
    ISBN 978-1-60714-424-3
  1. Chronic pain—Popular works. 2. Pain--Treatment—Popular works.
 I. Cleveland Clinic Foundation. II. Title. III. Title: Guide to pain management.
    RB127.S72765 2009
    616'.0472—dc22

                                                        2009026006

*This book is dedicated to the memory of
John J. Bonica, MD, the Italian physician who set
us on the path of recognizing and treating patients
with chronic intractable pain, thereby changing
the world forever. The information provided in this
text is also a testament to our patients and how
much they have taught us about their long-standing
symptoms, and how much we have yet to learn
regarding their palliation.*

*To my wife, Ursula, and my two sons,
Eric and Leif, whose attentions over the years were
compromised by my pursuit of pain medicine and
the acquisition of personal experience that forms
the basis of this book.*

Contents

Introduction

Pain has been a recorded part of the human vernacular since Babylonians and Sumerians carved their descriptions and treatments of pain on ancient stone tablets. Yet only recently have we made real strides in understanding and managing pain.

For centuries, pain, like illness, was blamed on external factors. Shamans and priestesses performed rites and ceremonies to battle demons and appease angry gods. In time, the Greeks and Romans came to believe that the brain and nervous system played a role in our perception of pain.

When medicine began to emerge as a science during the Renaissance, leading thinkers identified **acute pain as the body's response to harm.** Leonardo da Vinci and his peers perceived the brain as the seat of sensation and the spinal cord as the conduit through which sensation reached the brain.

It was not until the 17th century that French philosopher René Descartes proposed the model of the *pain pathway* that informs our view of pain today. Descartes saw the body as a machine and likened the pain pathway to the "bell-ringing mechanism in a church."

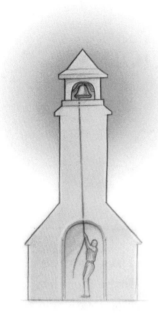

Just as pulling a rope at the bottom of a church tower triggers ringing in the bell high above, injuring one's foot, for example, triggers pain signals that Descartes depicted as "fast-moving particles of fire," creating a disturbance that "passes along the nerve filament until it reaches the brain."

Over time, we have coped with pain in various ways. The ancient Greeks and Incas bored holes in the skull to let pain escape. The Egyptians applied electric eels to painful wounds. Medieval practitioners used herbs and minerals to counteract pain. The 18th century saw the emergence of opiates, alcohol, and cocaine as therapies for pain. Laudanum, a combination of opium and alcohol, was a staple for treating pain and other illnesses in Victorian times. In the19th century, medical practitioners applied mustard plasters, quacks sold magnets, and researchers investigated pharmacological approaches (including anesthesia) that emerged as therapies for pain.

Awareness of pain has been amplified in recent decades, as we learn in ever greater detail about its origins, pathways, response to treatment—and prevalence.

We all experience a little more pain in our daily lives as we age, whether it's overall stiffness when we awaken or a longer recovery from intense physical activity. That is only natural. But pain is on the rise among Americans. The American Pain Foundation estimates that more than 50 million Americans suffer from chronic pain today, while only one in four receives proper pain treatment.

Often experience with pain begins with a benign injury or illness. Ankle sprains, broken toes, and grazed knees are common at any age. Typically, with rest and proper splinting, these injuries heal fairly quickly and the pain resolves. But if pain persists beyond three months, it can quickly become a monster that keeps us from working, sleeping, and otherwise engaging in life. It can worsen to the point that it dominates our every waking moment. Some people visit multiple doctors and endure untold procedures in an effort to cure their pain. They describe pain and its effects on their lives with vivid adjectives: *broken, shattered, robbed, chained, confined.*

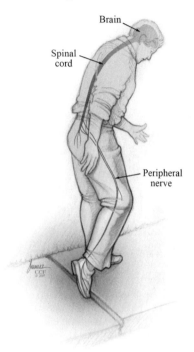

Despite the disability caused by chronic pain, the suffering it causes is often kept hidden. But the stories of some public figures who dealt privately with chronic pain have recently come to light. In 2002, the medical records of President John F. Kennedy were opened for research. Robert Dallek, a history professor at Boston University, and Jeffrey Kelman, MD, published *An Unfinished Life: John F. Kennedy, 1917–63*, detailing the late president's struggles with chronic pain.

"The lifelong health problems of John F. Kennedy constitute one of the best-kept secrets of recent U.S. history," wrote

Dallek later in the *Atlantic Monthly.* "Kennedy's charismatic appeal rested heavily on the image of youthful energy and good health he projected."

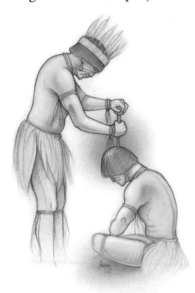

For thousands of years, man has coped with pain. Ancient Incas practiced trephination, *boring holes in the skull to let pain escape.*

But that vigor was a myth, Dallek wrote. Kennedy endured poking and prodding from many physicians from the time he was a boy. "God what a beating I'm taking," he wrote to a high school classmate. "All they do is talk about what an interesting case."

According to Dallek, "Kennedy was taking an extraordinary variety of medications: steroids for his Addison's disease; painkillers for his back; antispasmodics for his colitis; antibiotics for urinary-tract infections; antihistamines for allergies . . . ," as well as Nembutal to help him sleep. During his first senatorial campaign, he required crutches to make his way up flights of stairs. After campaigning, Kennedy would climb into the backseat of a car, "lean back . . . and close his eyes in pain," an aide recalled.

Kennedy wasn't the first president to suffer with a chronic health condition. Franklin Delano Roosevelt's struggle with polio failed to keep him from running the country. "Roosevelt, however, never needed the combination of medicines on which Kennedy relied to get through the day," wrote Dallek. Yet Kennedy convinced the American public—and indeed the world—that he was the picture of vitality. This reluctance to admit to suffering chronic pain persists even today. People with chronic pain are often stereotyped as being weak or hysterical, sometimes left to wonder if their pain is indeed in their imagination.

Writer and essayist Joan Didion wrote about her recurrent migraines in a 1968 essay entitled "In Bed," which was included in the 1990 collection of her work, *The White Album* (Farrar Straus and Giroux). She described spending one or two days a week almost unconscious with pain and deemed her suffering "a shameful secret."

But Didion shared a drive that many people with pain exhibit: a desire to regain control of their lives, a refusal to be defined by their pain alone. "I no longer fight. I lie down and let it happen," she wrote. And when the migraine pain receded, she emerged intact. "I open the windows and feel the air, eat gratefully, sleep well. I notice the particular nature of a flower in a glass on the stair landing. I count my blessings."

Chronic pain is exactly that—chronic. There is no magic bullet that will cure it. We have learned that a collaborative approach between physicians and specialists using a variety of approaches to manage chronic pain is most effective. As awareness grows among the members of the medical community about the causes and effects of pain, a wider effort is under way to educate both patients and primary-care physicians, who represent the front line in pain treatment, about its effective management.

This book looks at the disease process known as chronic pain. Case studies that describe the struggles of real people with pain will show how pain manifests in the body, what happens in specific pain conditions, and why the multidisciplinary approach to pain management is best.

Persistence is part of human nature. Despite physical limitations, mental strain, and a medical system less than well equipped to serve them, people with pain continue to hope and to advocate for themselves and others as they strive to recapture vitality in their lives.

Michael Stanton-Hicks, MB, BS, Dr. Med.
Cleveland Clinic

Chapter 1

What Is Chronic Pain?

We All Have Pain, But . . .

Everyone experiences pain. It's a necessary part of living. As our body's natural alarm system, pain alerts us when something goes wrong. Under normal circumstances, pain serves as a useful warning, our body's cry for help—similar to the squeal of an engine that runs dry of lubricant before seizing.

Stub a toe and the message travels instantly from the nerve ending in your foot to your spinal cord, where it is relayed to your brain. Within a split second, your mouth puts words to the pain: "Ouch!" Instinctively, you bend down to rub your toe and massage away the pain. If you've really whacked your toe, you may need to ice it to forestall swelling. For most of us, the pain dissipates in a few minutes, a few hours, or at worst a few days, and life goes on.

But for some, this tiny mishap eventually grows to such painful proportions that the mere movement of air across the toe sends daggers of pain shooting through the body. For the few who are unable to deactivate the body's constantly shrieking alarm system, the pain becomes chronic and develops into a disease process.

Phyllis

Pain had become a fact of life for Phyllis, a 40-year-old advertising executive. Her problems had begun a few years earlier, after she underwent surgery for acute back pain. The operation relieved her pain for a few months, but then she developed a dull, constant aching in her back. Pain sometimes shot down her left leg. Now her back pain was chronic.

Phyllis traveled frequently for work, and the cramped airline seats hurt her back. During the long presentations that were part of her life on the road, she was on her feet for hours at a time, in pain. It was something to be tolerated, to be dealt with later—in a long bath at the hotel, with some over-the-counter ibuprofen and perhaps a glass of wine. Unfortunately, Phyllis never slept well away from home, so she also popped a sleeping pill or two to avoid tossing and turning.

More often than not, Phyllis woke up stiff, sore, and occasionally groggy. Pulling herself together with a hot shower and a few cups of coffee, she ran for the airport, where the cycle began again.

Why Must Pain Be Treated if You Can Just "Grin and Bear It?"

Ignoring pain has serious consequences. Phyllis is one of the millions of Americans who press through their pain, never acknowledging the destruction it wreaks on their lives. They prefer to self-medicate rather than bother a doctor with their aches and pains. However, self-medication can have a disastrous effect when patients find they require increasingly strong doses of pain relievers, sleeping pills, and alcohol to dull their pain.

According to the American Pain Foundation, more than half of adults in the United States have experienced chronic or recurrent pain, and their numbers continue to increase. The impact of chronic pain is evident in all areas of society. Individuals under age 35 are about as likely as older Americans to experience pain. Chronic pain takes its greatest toll on working adults. Pain conditions cost workers more than four hours of productivity per week. That translates to economic losses of approximately $100 billion per year, but not because we are missing work. According to a 2003 report in the *Journal of the American Medical Association* (the most recent statistics available), nearly 80 percent of our lost productivity is explained by reduced work performance, not absenteeism.

Individuals such as Phyllis are probably unaware of the impact chronic pain has on the U.S. economy. But ignoring pain or self-medicating can lead to disaster on a more immediate level, too. For example, Phyllis earns a respectable salary and receives the added compensation of health and insurance benefits and a retirement plan. She has been dreaming about

Statistical Realities

- More than half the U.S. workforce reports regular head-aches, back pain, arthritis, or musculoskeletal pain.
- Two-thirds of the people living with chronic pain have done so for more than one year.
- One in three American adults loses more than 20 hours of sleep each month because of pain.
- Nearly three-quarters of current pain sufferers acknowledge that they've had to make adjustments in their lives.
- One-third of that group admits to making major life adjustments, including taking disability leave from work, changing jobs altogether, requiring assistance with activities of daily living, or moving to a home that is easier to manage.

purchasing a lakeside cottage. But if she becomes disabled by her pain, she faces a loss of income, further surgery, months of rehabilitation, emotional distress, and the restriction of tennis, golf, and long-distance travel. If her pain goes untreated, it may increase with age, making it impossible for her to participate in those water-based activities that she most wants to enjoy while she resides at her lake house.

As people succumb to the realities of pain-related disability, they often find themselves sinking into depression. Many studies have shown that, in an increasingly desperate search for relief, many patients may contemplate swallowing even more pain pills—to end their pain once and for all.

Downplaying Pain in America

Americans downplay pain as an annoying side effect or a natural consequence of aging. A recent survey found that we rank pain as least problematic on a list of health concerns that includes cancer, obesity, heart disease, alcohol and drug abuse, and AIDS.

But chronic pain is a bona fide disease that is on the rise. This can be explained in part by cultural changes that have occurred over the past century. Americans have moved from a life that once involved hard physical activity to more sedentary occupations. As we migrated from the countryside to the city, our lives became less physically active. In place of physical activity, we have gained increased stress, dysfunctional muscles, poor sleep quality, and poor nutrition. Our reliance on convenience and labor-saving devices has exacerbated the problem.

This lifestyle is the perfect recipe for developing conditions that lead to chronic muscular pain. Nearly 70 percent of painful conditions suffered by Americans arise from muscle dysfunction. The numbers are much lower in individuals, such as farmers, whose musculature is well developed from a lifetime of strenuous physical activity. Further complicating the matter is the failure of many physicians to acknowledge chronic pain. Only in relatively recent times has the field of pain management earned recognition as a medical specialty. Because most physicians have never been taught the difference between acute and chronic pain, their treatment approach is often the same for both conditions.

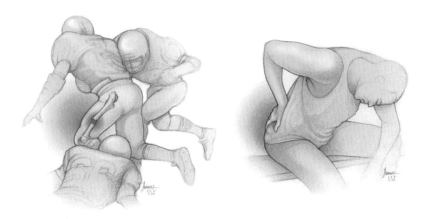

Chronic pain (right) does not respond well to measures used for acute pain (left).

But the truth is that therapies for acute pain cannot adequately address the interrelated components—physical, psychological, pharmacological, and therapeutic—of chronic pain.

Even a simple injury can bring unending pain. One misstep changed the life of 56-year-old Bob forever.

Bob

In a bout of spring cleaning, Bob was helping his wife clear out the basement when he tripped on the stairs, sustaining what appeared to be a simple broken ankle. The bones were set, he was fitted with a cast, and he figured he'd be off his crutches in six weeks. Three months later, Bob was still in agony.

In 90 percent of patients, a broken ankle will heal in less than three months, with pain dissipating more rapidly. But in the remainder, the broken bone may be accompanied by a nerve injury. And nervous system damage is the bedrock of chronic pain. In Bob's case, when his ankle was set, the tibial nerve (which runs down the back of the leg to the ankle) was injured. The inflamed nerve became entrapped within its narrow tunnel in the ankle. Pain, burning, and tingling set in, in a condition called tarsal tunnel syndrome, akin to carpal tunnel syndrome in the wrist.

But Bob's problems didn't stop there. His entire leg changed color, swelled, and became exquisitely sensitive to light, touch, air movement, and cold temperatures. His symptoms became consuming, occurring relentlessly all day and all night. At this stage, the only means of controlling Bob's incessant pain was a multidisciplinary approach that combined medication and local anesthesia, rehabilitation, psychological help, and continued reassurance of recovery.

Bob's tarsal tunnel syndrome evolved into complex regional pain syndrome, or CRPS (further described in chapter 4). Doctors now believe that certain people may have a genetic predisposition to CRPS, in which the normal physiology of the nervous system is disturbed. Pain signals are no longer sent solely from the site of injury. Instead, they spread.

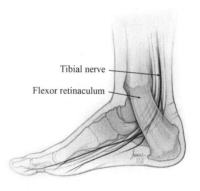

Tibial nerve
Flexor retinaculum

For Bob, an accident resulting from a simple Saturday chore led to a syndrome that left him severely debilitated, unable to work or to help around the house. When Bob's broken ankle was set, the tibial nerve was injured. The inflamed nerve became entrapped within its narrow channel. Pain, burning, and tingling set in—a condition called tarsal tunnel syndrome.

The Desperate Search for Pain Relief

Patients with chronic pain offer sharply detailed descriptions of their pain, often describing it as "burning," "like being stabbed with a hot poker," or "knifelike." As a first step, they typically try to cope with their pain using nonsteroidal anti-inflammatory drugs or NSAIDS, such as Tylenol (acetaminophen) or Advil (ibuprofen). When patients such as Bob return to their orthopedist with complaints of persistent pain from a fracture, sprain, or strain, they are usually referred back to their primary-care physician. Internists and family physicians typically manage the pain by prescribing medications from the family of anti-inflammatory drugs. But eventually these drugs may not prove to be strong enough. So the physicians may prescribe Darvocet (propoxyphene napsylate and acetaminophen) or Tylenol (acetaminophen) with codeine to alleviate the patient's pain. Then, when these medications no longer help, they turn to stronger medications, perhaps prescribing opiates (narcotics derived from opium) such as OxyContin (oxycodone).

As a patient's tolerance of opiates increases, a good primary-care physician will become concerned. Abuse of prescription narcotics is on the rise, and the U.S. Drug Enforcement Agency, which grants prescribing privileges to physicians, is actively cracking down on the problem. The notoriety surrounding the few who became addicted to prescription narcotics has led to an increase in DEA raids on doctors' offices and brought pharmacists under pressure to report excessive doses of prescription narcotics. In 2004, the DEA reversed its support of guidelines for narcotics prescription that had been negotiated with pain-management specialists. This reversal dealt a blow to the practice of pain management, particularly at the end of life. Increased policing measures fail to account for the fact that patients with chronic pain are often profoundly undertreated—the reason that some states have approved "Compassionate Care" bills, which relax the rules governing the prescription of opiates for chronic pain.

But the reversal has led to other unintended consequences as well. On January 10, 2006, Jane E. Brody wrote in the *New York Times*, "The growing number of arrests of pain-management specialists is exacting high costs for patients, physicians, and medical insurers. Some doctors order costly but unnecessary diagnostic tests so they can show the DEA a reason for prescribing strong pain medication."

When patients with chronic pain are denied prescriptions, they may become angry and elect to "take their business elsewhere." In doing so, they often endure stereotyping as doctor-shoppers or pill-poppers. But in our experience, there is a profound dichotomy between pain management and society's labeling of people with chronic pain as hypochondriacal, weak, or needing training in anger management. Unfortunately, the problem is equally pervasive inside the medical community, in large part because pain management is such a young field.

Unfortunately, when patients in chronic pain watch the local ranks of supportive physicians and pharmacists—their sources for pain relief—dwindle, they can become desperate.

My Pain Problem As "Mind Over Matter"— Can't I Control It through Mental Discipline?

Phyllis and Bob share a unique American attribute when it comes to chronic pain: like many of us, they assumed that positive thinking could overcome their pain. A 2003 national survey found that an overwhelming 84 percent of adults believe that our state of mind influences our experience of physical pain, suggesting that pain can be controlled by the mind alone.

Yet chronic pain often does not resolve, despite expectations to the contrary. It's true that some of us are far less prone than others to complain about pain and to seek relief from it. The reasons? We may have a high tolerance for pain, we may be naturally stoic, or we may prefer to avoid medications because of their side effects. The truth is, chronic pain affects all personality types.

Fortunately, there are ways to lessen the severity of pain symptoms and to dramatically improve the quality of life for people who suffer from chronic pain. These involve a multifaceted approach that encompasses medical, psychological, and even alternative therapies. If such measures are adopted early enough, they provide relief for a high percentage of patients, allowing them to function much more normally.

Dispelling the Myths About Pain

Chronic pain and its treatments are steeped in myth. Some of the common beliefs held by people who develop chronic pain or by the well-meaning relatives or friends who advise them will be addressed. Additionally, there is a lack of understanding and reluctance to accept that pain may persist in spite of all medical measures.

Is Pain a Natural Side Effect of Aging?

As people age, some "nuisance pain" resulting from physical wear and tear is natural. The cartilage that cushions our joints may deteriorate over time, along with the disks that cushion the vertebrae in our spine. Some loss of suppleness is to be expected. Aging creates a double whammy, however, when we add chronic pain to the mixture.

Chronic pain worsens over time, although to what degree is unpredictable and depends upon many unknowns. Most chronic pain results in loss of function in the neck, back, or extremities; less frequently, it affects the face or head. If pain causes us to protect a painful neck, back, arm, or leg by not using it, then we can expect a loss of function in the affected joints, muscles, and surrounding structures, much as an athlete on the disabled list loses muscle conditioning. With disuse, blood supply to the area is reduced and arthritis can set in, further increasing our pain and discomfort. Conversely, activity restores circulation, which is good for the bones and joints.

To preserve optimal function and sustain vitality, activity levels should be gradually increased through a supervised rehabilitation program. The goal of living with chronic pain is not to cure it, but to manage it.

I've Heard that I Shouldn't Exercise if I'm in Pain Because I Could Further Injure Myself. Is This True?

No. In fact, exercise via physical therapy can be key to successful rehabilitation. When we don't use our muscles, they atrophy, literally shrinking in size. Some chronic-pain patients understand this and comply with prescribed exercises; some resist exercising and inadvertently become their own worst enemies.

Just as a good coach can make or break a team, a good physical or occupational therapist can have a dramatic impact on pain. Much of what is provided during physical therapy is encouragement—reassurance that initial discomfort is not harmful, but is in fact necessary to regain function. If, however, pain is so severe that exercise is prevented, then anesthesiologists can insert a catheter and administer a local anesthetic that will block pain signals from reaching the affected area. This is almost guaranteed to help patients over that first big bump in the road to rehabilitation.

Physical and occupational therapists also address avoidance or *guarding* behaviors that are often observed during the acute phase of injury (see page 89 for a more in-depth discussion of this phenomenon). Guarding spurs a vicious cycle during which attempts at physical activity increase pain, essentially punishing patients for their efforts to engage in activity. As the cycle progresses, patients becomes less mobile and more socially withdrawn, which reinforces their view of themselves as disabled.

A note about workers' compensation and related litigation: these processes can become impediments to successful pain management when patients who rely on or anticipate income from a work-related injury knowingly or unknowingly resist recovery.

Can I Become Addicted to Painkillers If I Take Them for Too Long?

To put it bluntly, the risk of addiction is exaggerated. The incidence of narcotic addiction among chronic-pain patients is about the same as in the general population: 6 percent. This means that only 3 in every 1,000 patients succumb to addiction.

Although pain-management specialists share this data with patients and families, we find ourselves continually having to reassure patients that the use of narcotics is essential if they are to recover from disability.

In fact, we have learned that when doses of pain medications are less than adequate—which is often the case in the United States—then patients risk developing *pseudo-addiction.* This is not the drug-seeking behavior of addicts or of dealers hoping to sell prescription narcotics on the street. Rather, pseudo-addiction is the relief-seeking behavior of patients in pain, who will stop asking for more medication once they receive the proper dose of narcotic.

A trial-and-error period of adjustment to these medications is important, particularly for patients with neuropathic pain who may require more than one medication. The goal is to find the dose that works best for the pain without causing other problems, which can range from sedation and sleepiness to depression, ringing in the ears, and even psychotic behaviors.

In rare instances, opiate addiction can develop. One expert who treats patients with chronic pain and addiction says that he has frequently come upon the myth that "an addictive personality makes you susceptible to addiction because you're needy, weak, or immoral."

However, he points out, "Addiction is not necessarily a result of a character deficit or personality flaw. It's a disease, and it's genetic."

The vast majority of people who become addicted to painkillers have a history of substance abuse. There are three criteria that define addiction, and most chronic-pain patients demonstrate the first two: increased tolerance for and physical dependence upon a substance. Pain patients know they have an addiction when they develop what one doctor calls the *Three Cs:*

- Compulsion and/or craving for the medication
- Loss of control
- Continued use of the medication despite adverse consequences

In these cases, it is surprising to learn that those who suffer from alcoholism as well as chronic pain can handle opioid therapy quite well. In contrast, people who have been recreational drug users or have had specific narcotic addictions in the past do poorly with opioids. As we are now learning, addiction is a disease process, most likely genetically based.

Will I Have a Heart Attack if I Take a COX-2 Inhibitor for My Pain?

In 2004, a storm of controversy erupted around the COX-2 inhibitors such as Vioxx, Celebrex, and Bextra. Because these drugs may cause heart or vascular problems, both Vioxx and Bextra were withdrawn from the market in spite of being very effective anti-inflammatory (rheumatologic) medications.

The truth is that these problems occur in just a fraction of patients and that the benefits of COX-2 inhibitors for people in chronic pain may well outweigh their risks. Patients who do not do well on NSAIDs, such as ibuprofen or acetaminophen, often find very low doses of Celebrex—the only COX-2 inhibitor currently available in the United States—to be very helpful.

It is true that the undesirable side effects of pain-relieving medications may become clear only after years or decades of the drugs being in use. But physicians who specialize in pain management are well aware of the drugs' shortcomings and side effects. That is why the drugs are prescribed with discretion and accompanied by frequent monitoring. Blood tests at regular intervals provide early warnings of potential damage to the kidney or liver, the organs that process drugs in the body.

The COX-2 inhibitor debate was tinged with an air of hysteria, but it is worthwhile to discuss the risks and benefits of these drugs seriously with your physician. In particular, patients must make their physicians aware of any other medical issues they have, in addition to chronic pain (such as vascular or heart disease), that may influence the choice of medication.

Can Chronic Pain Kill Me?

Chronic pain can't kill you, but it can have a profound impact on your quality of life. It all depends on how your body deals with pain and how committed you are to managing your pain. There is no quick fix for chronic pain, but there are many options.

Some chronic pain, such as the pain associated with shingles (post-herpetic neuralgia), can interfere with a person's overall sense of well-being. Situations like Henry's, described in chapter 3, can prompt suicidal feelings when pain seems unbearable and a normal life completely out of reach.

Actor and comedian Jerry Lewis offers another example. His trademark pratfalls took an excruciating toll on his body, leading to nearly four decades of chronic back pain, countless doctor visits, and years of addiction to prescription narcotics. Today, Lewis speaks frequently about his experiences with chronic pain and credits his young daughter with saving his life when she found him, suicidal, with a gun in hand. Now without pain, he is equally grateful to the pain team that permanently implanted a neurostimulator in his spine. Advocating for passage of a national pain-care policy before a group of legislators in September 2005, Lewis said that he was reengaged in life and was remastering the old movies in which he starred with Dean Martin.

Can I Make My Pain Worse by Giving In to It?

Physical pain is real. As explained in chapter 3, pain signals are transmitted along nerve pathways when tissue is damaged or when the nervous system misfires. But the psychological suffering connected to physical pain is very much in our minds.

Perhaps the hardest part of learning to live with residual pain is learning not to suffer with it. It is the management of it, rather than its cure, that should be the goal of patients who suffer from chronic pain.

Both Hinduism and Buddhism have much to teach us on this subject. These religions teach that human suffering is part of life and that suffering is broken down into outer conditions and inner responses. In chronic pain, the painful stimulus represents the outer condition. The inner responses, or the way we interpret that stimulus, take place in the mind.

Obviously, we have little control over outer conditions such as the fall in the hockey rink that fractures an ankle and leads to complex regional pain syndrome, but most of us have the capacity to control our inner responses. It is inner control that can be developed in the context of a multidisciplinary pain program. The team's neurologist, anesthesiologist, rheumatologist, physical and occupational therapists, psychologist, and pain nurses each contributes his or her expertise so patients with difficult pain conditions can learn to experience the minimal amount of pain. All aspects of your pain are addressed: its cause, if still present; the systems affected (joints, muscles, blood vessels, nerves); and pain behaviors.

The Placebo Effect. The renowned physician Sir William Osler observed that "the desire to take medicine is perhaps the greatest feature that distinguishes man from animals."

Considering the nature of the nostrums humankind has employed over the centuries, another distinguishing characteristic is our ability to survive medicine! It is a well-known medical phenomenon that about 35 percent of patients will respond positively to placebos—treatments that have no effect. In a pioneering University of Michigan Health System study reported in 2005, researchers were able to directly link the brain's pain-fighting chemicals (endorphins) to the placebo effect and to a corresponding decrease in pain levels. This study begins to explain why so many people claim relief from therapies that have no real physical benefit—and why cognitive and behavioral therapies can so effectively manage chronic pain.

A final consideration with respect to pain and the power of the mind: the mental imagery that patients use to describe their pain is highly revealing. We hear descriptions such as "the pain is stabbing me in the eyes with knitting needles" or

The Pain Is His (or Her) Problem, Not Mine

Each human being reacts to pain differently. We may be stoic or quite vocal about our discomfort; and we may react to pain suffered by family members in different ways. It is, therefore, important for the pain team to understand how families respond to the problems of pain patients.

Sometimes family members may claim that the patient is exaggerating symptoms as a ploy to gain attention. This can trigger family dysfunction or marital discord, or exaggerate preexisting problems. Sometimes a spouse uses pain to justify the avoidance of intimacy. In these cases, it's important to determine whether a problem in the relationship is perpetuating the chronic pain state and sabotaging rehabilitation efforts.

Equally counterproductive to functional recovery—particularly in the setting of chronic pain—is reinforcement of the patient's sick role by family members. As pain specialists, we try to identify aspects of the patient's pain and disability that are reinforced by family members, who may be completely unaware of their actions in order to maximize rehabilitation measures.

"the pain feels like a thousand knives passing through my leg." While the pain is real, these images serve only to emphasize and exaggerate the experience of pain.

Now that you know what chronic pain is and is not, let's take a look at the gains in the medical field of pain management. Quite apart from the significant developments in pharmaceuticals, international techniques, and genetics is the acceptance that good pain management requires a multidisciplinary or multispeciality approach to achieve optimal results.

Chapter 2

The Evolution of Pain Management

"Chronic pain disables more people than cancer or heart disease and it costs the American people more money than both." —John Bonica, MD

In 1944, during World War II, a 27-year-old army doctor named John Bonica was assigned to Fort Lewis in Tacoma, Washington. Bonica was named chief of anesthesiology at Madigan Army Hospital, one of the largest American military hospitals of the time, with 7,700 beds. Madigan was also one of the two largest debarkation hospitals

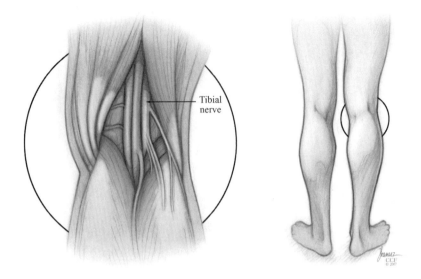

A popliteal nerve block induces analgesia in branches of the sciatic nerve for diagnosis and pain relief in the leg and foot.

on the West Coast, receiving thousands of wounded military personnel from overseas. At the understaffed hospital, Bonica was responsible for the care of more than 10,000 soldiers who had been wounded in the Pacific theater of operations. The young doctor was charged with providing anesthesia prior to surgery and with managing patients who had severe pain or pulmonary problems.

The job was overwhelming. Time was short, the patients kept coming, and trained physicians and nurse anesthetists were scarce. Bonica anesthetized more than 50 patients each day for their operations. The vast experience he accrued with various forms of anesthesia taught him a great deal about regional anesthetic techniques such as nerve blocks. (Regional blocks numb only those nerves providing sensation to a specific area of the body.)

At times abrupt with hospital staff, Bonica was a dedicated and compassionate caregiver when it came to his patients' well-being. His experimentation with nerve blocks spurred a lifelong crusade to understand why so many patients developed intractable pain long after injuries or illnesses resolved— and a search for the Holy Grail of pain relief.

Bonica was quick to share his knowledge, initiating a training program for physicians and nurse anesthetists who were assigned to forward hospitals in the combat zones of the Pacific theater of operations. In the spring of 1945, with the support of the surgeon general, Bonica published the first comprehensive treatise on anesthesiology. The addition of trained staff at Madigan allowed Bonica to concentrate on treating patients with severely painful injuries—those he felt were being neglected in the crush of medical emergencies.

Soldiers with Lingering Pain

According to UCLA Biomedical Library archives, Bonica reported encountering cases that baffled him. Long after their bones had healed and their nerves had regenerated, soldiers who had undergone amputation reported pain in missing limbs and a variety of obscure neurological and musculoskeletal symptoms.

Bonica decided to tackle the problem of phantom pain (discussed in further detail in chapter 4). With few answers available in the scientific literature of the time, Bonica sent the soldiers for consultations with colleagues: an orthopedic specialist, a neurosurgeon, and a psychiatrist. "They knew less than I did," he reported.

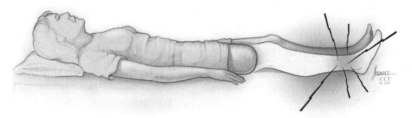

Phantom pain is felt at the site of the original pain.

Bonica realized that little information existed about the treatment of chronic pain because little research had been done on pain itself. Furthermore, the meager knowledge that did exist was not accessible to the practicing physician, scattered as it was through innumerable books and journals. As a result, the average physician knew little if anything about the basic principles of managing chronic pain. Finally, Bonica saw that the treatment of complex pain problems required vast knowledge and experience—much more than any one individual could accrue under normal circumstances.

To reduce the suffering of patients with chronic pain, Bonica came up with a creative plan. He instituted twice-weekly meetings with colleagues in psychiatry, orthopedics, and neurology, believing that collaboration was key to understanding chronic pain and how to treat it. Word of Bonica's work spread, and upon his discharge as a major in 1946, he joined the staff at Tacoma General Hospital to put his theory of multidisciplinary pain management into practice. There, Bonica founded the world's first true multidisciplinary pain center.

Bringing Pain Management to the Masses

At Tacoma General, Bonica's focus turned toward obstetric pain after his wife, Emma, nearly died during the birth of their first child. Obstetricians of the era relied on ether anesthesia to relieve labor pains. Bonica was convinced that regional anesthesia would be safer and more effective. Emma Bonica later became the first woman in the Pacific Northwest to receive the continuous epidural anesthesia routinely used in childbirth today.

Bonica's early work primarily impacted pain management in army hospitals and hospitals in the Pacific Northwest, but by 1950 he had accumulated enough data on more

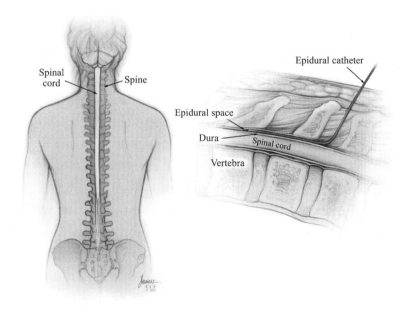

Continuous epidural anesthesia is achieved through the insertion of a small catheter in the spine as show above (right).

than 2,000 patients to begin writing what would become the bible of pain diagnosis and therapy for physicians worldwide. His 1,500-page book, *The Management of Pain,* was first published in 1953. The massive text challenged the health-care industry to find solutions for acute and chronic pain. It called for multidisciplinary management, recognizing that no single specialty offered expertise in all the nuances of chronic pain. Bonica published a similarly comprehensive companion book, *Principles and Practices of Obstetric Analgesia and Anesthesia,* in 1967, and an updated edition of *The Management of Pain* in 1990, four years before his death.

A Growing Field

The field of pain management gained tremendous momentum during the 1970s. Patients worldwide were referred to Bonica's revolutionary pain clinic, eventually prompting him to organize the first international symposium on pain management in 1973. Convening for this event, clinicians, scientists, health-care workers, and representatives of state and federal institutions (including the National Institutes of Health) met in a monastery in Providence Heights, Washington.

The symposium's enthusiastic reception prompted the creation of the International Association for the Study of Pain (IASP), which promotes research and education into the causes and treatment of chronic pain. In 1977, the American Pain Society (APS) was formed, launching the *Journal of Pain,* now considered the most prestigious and ground-breaking peer-reviewed scientific journal on pain research and practice. During that decade, major inroads were made into the understanding of pain. In one advance, researchers pinpointed the sites responding to tissue injury in the peripheral nervous system (the network of nerves that transmit messages from other parts of the body to the brain and spinal cord) and the central nervous system (the brain and spinal cord).

Bonica worked tirelessly to educate the public and the government about the immense costs of acute and chronic pain for our society. Joining him in this crusade were nurses who had long been advocates for effective management of patients' pain. The issue resonated deeply with the public as well as with members of Congress. Bonica eventually found the ear of the U.S. Agency for Healthcare Policy and Research (AHCPR). Following extensive government hearings, in 1989 pain management earned official recognition in U.S. health-care practice. But getting effective treatment for chronic pain remained difficult, a situation complicated by the failure of insurance companies to cover the costs of pain management. Fortunately, the last decade has seen extensive progress in this arena, as insurers increasingly recognize the long-term financial impact of not covering treatment for chronic pain and as grant monies become available for research into effective therapies.

Today, Bonica's multidisciplinary approach to pain has been widely adopted and even expanded. Physical therapy, biofeedback (behavioral training in which patients learn to control physiological responses), and even integrative therapies such as hypnosis and acupuncture are now common components of pain management. Pain management is one of the fastest growing subspecialties in medicine today, yet the need to raise awareness of pain and pain management persists. Medical schools still do not incorporate pain management into the curriculum of primary-care physicians, and Americans still seek pharmaceutical salvation in that one magical cure-all drug. Education about pain management begins with an understanding of pain itself, how it manifests in our bodies, and how it can be measured.

Chapter 3

The Nervous System and Pain

I n order to understand pain and where it comes from, it's important to understand the nervous system.

How Does the Body Process Pain Messages?

Think of your nervous system as an elaborate communication device composed of your brain and spinal cord (central nervous system), as well as the network of sensory and motor nerves that transmit messages from every other part of your body back to your brain and spinal cord (peripheral nervous system).

Peripheral nerves vary in size and send signals through the spinal cord to the brain at varying rates. The smallest peripheral nerve fibers are called nociceptors, and they are found by

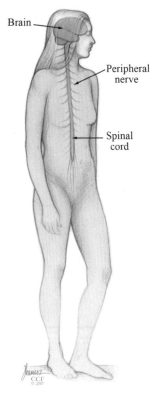

the millions in skin, bones, joints, muscles, and protective membranes around our organs. Nociceptors respond to temperature, vibration, pressure, and even the lightest touch. It is the nociceptors that sense tissue damage and send pain signals to the spinal cord.

Severe pain rushes messages from nociceptors in the peripheral nervous system to the central nervous system. The spinal cord receives these signals and then releases chemical messengers (neurotransmitters) that travel to the brain, where the information is processed.

The thalamus, a collection of cells at the base of the brain, is the most important way station for all types of pain impulses arising from every region of the body. This structure not only receives this information, but it integrates, modifies, and prioritizes the pain impulses via connections to one of three specialized regions of the brain:

- The somatosensory cortex, which processes information about physical sensations
- The limbic system, which processes information about feelings and emotions
- The frontal cortex, which processes information involving thought

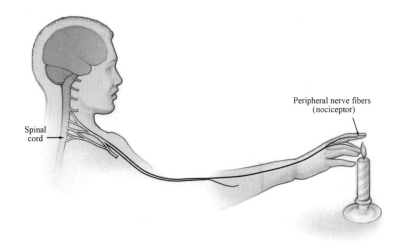

Spinal cord

Peripheral nerve fibers (nociceptor)

Nociceptors respond to temperature, vibration, pressure, and even the lightest touch. It is the nociceptors that sense tissue damage and send pain signals to the spinal cord.

Two Kinds of Chronic Pain

There are two types of chronic pain: nociceptive pain and neuropathic pain. *Nociceptive pain* is triggered by tissue damage, usually involving sprains, fractures, burns, bumps, or bruises. Nociceptors become irritated when bones, muscles, or joints are injured or overused. Patients describe throbbing or a dull aching that normally resolves with rest and NSAIDS. In a short time, the tissue heals and pain disappears.

Nociceptive pain is also triggered by internal organs, such as the heart, stomach, appendix, or bladder. In these cases, the pain a patient feels is called *visceral pain*. This type of nociceptive pain can be difficult to pinpoint, with dull, vague, sporadic pains radiating away from their source. Nociceptive pain can become chronic when conditions such as arthritis

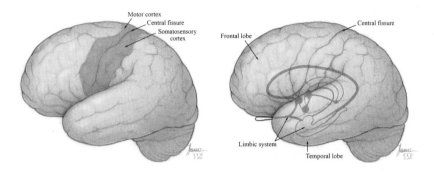

The figures above show two important areas in the brain, the somatosensory cortex (left) and the limbic system (right), where pain impulses are processed.

create constant joint irritation or conditions such as cancer produce constant visceral pain.

In contrast, *neuropathic pain* is triggered by damage to nerves or by nervous system dysfunction, and it may last much longer. Pain caused by nerve damage is seen in peripheral neuropathy arising from diabetes or other conditions, as well as in carpal tunnel or tarsal tunnel syndromes, which entrap the nerves. Nervous system dysfunction is seen in complex regional pain syndrome and phantom pain, where the brain distorts ordinary sensations or misinterprets them as pain signals.

Both types of pain heighten the body's sensitivity to pain. The nociceptors fire with unusual intensity, amplifying pain signals far out of proportion to the actual problem. By way of comparison, think of music being blasted through a stereo, or of a shrieking alarm jolting you from sleep. The pain signals continue to fire long after an acute problem has healed.

Researchers are just beginning to understand what is happening in the body when a patient experiences neuropathic pain. Investigations are focusing on proteins in the

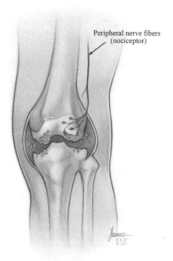

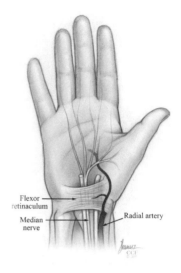

Chronic arthritis: Nociceptors become irritated when bones and joints are injured or overused (nociceptive pain).

Carpal tunnel syndrome: Nerves become damaged by being entrapped (neuropathic pain).

brain that trigger changes in nerve cells that, in turn, amplify and sustain our response to pain. In addition, according to research funded by the National Institutes of Health, there is increasing evidence suggesting that some of us have a genetic predisposition to the development of chronic pain.

Confounding research into chronic pain is the fact that pain signals and pain tolerance are affected by a host of outside factors, including:

- Emotional and psychological well-being
- Social and cultural influences
- Age and gender
- Attitude and expectations
- Past pain experiences

The following case study exemplifies how the combination of nociceptive and neuropathic pain over a long period causes the pain experience to become amplified by changes in the nervous system.

Jane

Jane was in her mid-50s when she slipped on the ice outside her home and injured her shoulder. The injury eventually healed, but her shoulder remained painful, and her doctors noticed a gradual deterioration in shoulder function. They recommended a shoulder replacement to correct the problem. But Jane was terrified of surgery. At the time, shoulder-replacement surgery was not nearly as common as knee- and hip-replacement surgery. Also, she was unconvinced that surgery would eliminate her shoulder pain. Not satisfied that surgery was worth the risk, Jane decided against it.

Fast-forward 20 years. Jane is now in her mid-70s and in frail health. Over the past two decades, she has resorted to innumerable over-the-counter and prescription narcotics to manage her pain. She pops Nuprin, an over-the-counter form of ibuprofen, by the fistful. But her self-medication routine has damaged the lining of her stomach, creating a bleeding ulcer that required surgery.

Jane's primary-care physician prescribed Percocet (oxycodone and acetaminophen) for her shoulder pain. As her tolerance for the narcotic increased, so did her intake. Jane's body was absorbing more and more of the narcotic, rendering it less effective. It is natural for pain patients to build up a tolerance of prescription narcotics and to require more than the average person. However,

prescribing physicians can find the increasing dosage star-
tling and become wary of drawing unwarranted DEA
attention. Jane's doctor grew reluctant to prescribe Perco-
cet at such high levels and frequency.

One day, Jane accidentally overdosed on her Perco-
cet—an event not uncommon among elderly patients.
She was hospitalized and forced to endure detoxification,
even though her medication had been prescribed. The
attending physicians flagged her as a geriatric psychiatric
patient. With such high levels of narcotics in her system,
they assumed that Jane had attempted suicide. Jane's
family struggled to convince numerous doctors that Jane
had accidentally taken more of her high dose of prescrip-
tion medication than necessary and that she was not at
risk for suicide.

Eventually, the family decided that the best route for
managing Jane's pain was to manage her prescriptions.
So her children took turns delivering doses morning and
night to ensure that Jane wouldn't take too much medica-
tion. They undertook this burden willingly to ensure her
health and safety.

What Causes Peripheral Neuropathy?

Damage to the peripheral nervous system—which subsequently can cause pain—is most often caused by high glucose
levels, which can produce chemical changes in the nerves that
interfere with their signaling ability. However, chronic alcohol use, exposure to toxins (including chemotherapy drugs),
vitamin deficiency, and a host of other health problems can
also trigger peripheral neuropathy. *Neuropathy* is a term

describing pathological changes in nerves, frequently leading to chronic pain.

Neuropathy can also be a symptom of shingles, or post-herpetic neuralgia. Shingles is caused by reactivation of the chickenpox virus (*varicella zoster*) long after an episode of infection has occurred, typically in childhood. The chickenpox virus doesn't disappear; instead, it lies dormant in the nerve roots, often for decades. Typically, a weakened immune system paves the way for shingles to occur, such as in the case of Henry.

Henry

Like most people of his generation, Henry suffered through a bout of chickenpox as a youngster. Now in his 80s, he has been lonely and depressed since the death of his wife a few months ago. He isn't sleeping well, and he has put nutrition on the back burner, making do with canned soup and frozen dinners.

Fatigue and poor nutrition have weakened his immune system. He developed a bad case of influenza, followed by pain across his chest. Henry was too depressed to seek help, even when an excruciatingly painful band of chickenpox-like blisters appeared on his chest. The blisters turned into scars, but the pain remained just as intense. Because the pain became unbearable, he finally sought medical help from his local practitioner, but none of the medications the doctor prescribed did anything to relieve his pain. Henry was finally referred to pain management specialists who used a variety of medicines and techniques to improve his pain control. The condition Henry was enduring—called post-herpetic neuralgia—can be so severe that if uncontrolled it can cause patients to take their lives. There were times when Henry contemplated suicide as a viable option to end his pain.

Henry is not alone; the risk of developing shingles is 70 percent among Americans over age 80 and even higher after age 90. Weakened immunity, compounded by the stress of major losses and life changes, increases the susceptibility of senior citizens to shingles. However, shingles need not herald the onset of neuropathic pain. Prompt treatment with anti-viral medication can limit nerve damage, speed healing, and prevent peripheral neuropathy.

Can Chronic Pain Be Cured?

One big difference between chronic conditions and acute illnesses is that a chronic condition generally requires life-long management. Unlike an acute injury or illness, which has a definite beginning and end, chronic neuropathic pain endures, although with proper medication your feelings of discomfort may be significantly lessened. Opioids are less effective in treating neuropathic pain than they are in treating acute pain. But other drugs such as anti-epilepsy medicines and antidepressants may be helpful. Even though pain may not be fully reversible for patients such as Jane and Henry, treatment can lessen its severity and allow them to enjoy a more vibrant life. It should also be said that it is not uncommon for an identifiable cause of pain to be discovered during a patient's clinical evaluation, in which case whatever means are necessary are then deployed to remove or treat the underlying problem.

Questions for Your Primary Care Doctor

- Do you understand the kind of pain I feel?
- Do I need to see a specialist for my pain?
- Will pain medicine help me?
- Does the pain medication have side effects?
- Am I at risk of seizures from the pain medication?
- Do I need other medication to manage any side effects?
- Can I become addicted to my pain medication?
- How often should I take my pain medicine?
- Is it safe to take over-the-counter pain relievers as well?
- What other steps can I take to manage my pain?

When the Nervous System Misfires

Nociceptive pain usually becomes chronic only with constant tissue irritation. At times, however, the nervous system misfires. Some patients may be predisposed to the development of nociceptive pain because of what is described as *sensitization* in the central nervous system. This type of pain may also have a neuropathic component, suggesting that some nerve damage may have occurred as a result of an injury, as happened in John's case.

John

John is what you'd call a weekend warrior. He tries to exercise regularly, but at age 43 he finds that his job as a sales manager and his responsibilities as a father of two make that difficult, except for on weekends. During a particularly intense game of basketball in the driveway one Saturday, John turned his ankle. Doctors diagnosed a sprain. He was told that with early treatment and adequate rest, it should heal within a few weeks.

But three months after his mishap, John's ankle was still throbbing. He could no longer participate in any kind of exercise, and the pain began to have an impact on his sleep, family life, and work. John's internal alarm system was malfunctioning, screeching at ever-higher decibels. His nociceptive pain had become chronic, and his attempts to cope with it only caused additional suffering as he tried to "drink the pain away."

John's wife eventually convinced him to seek help from a pain specialist. He received a sympathetic-nerve block, an injection of anesthetic to modify pain signals from his ankle and prevent them from traveling first to the spinal cord and from there to his brain. This provided some physical relief. John also began taking an antidepressant to alleviate the depression brought on by his pain. In addition, he learned better coping mechanisms, thanks to psychological counseling he received as part of his pain-management plan. John also began to attend Alcoholics Anonymous meetings.

Though he has not resumed his weekend basketball games, John is tackling his outdoor chores and enjoying his children, thanks to a comprehensive approach to his pain.

The only constant in the human experience of pain is that intensity of sensation and levels of tolerance are unique to each individual, although specific pain entities bring with them specific characteristics, management, and outcomes.

Chapter 4

Navigating Chronic Pain

C hronic pain manifests in myriad ways. Sometimes, large areas of the body are affected. At other times, pain zeroes in on key targets, such as the big toe. In pain syndromes (aggregates of symptoms that occur simultaneously), whole regions and several systems in the body may be affected. Furthermore, the causes of pain are diverse. Here are some of the most common and most notable compass points in the vast territory we know as chronic pain.

Arthritis

Jack, age 40, played football throughout high school and college. The stance required during his years of play and practice has left both knees painful and stiff to the point of beginning to hobble him. Arthritis is one of the most common chronic health problems in our society. An umbrella term for more than 100 diseases that target our joints and musculoskeletal system, *arthritis* produces joint pain, stiffness, inflammation, and in some cases deformity. Bones, tendons, and ligaments are affected, along with surrounding muscles. This can make simple tasks such as tying a shoe, opening a jar, or walking across a room extremely difficult.

The Arthritis Foundation reports that 43 million Americans have physician-diagnosed arthritis and another 23 million suffer chronic joint symptoms. Women are twice as likely as men to develop some form of arthritis, and baby boomers will soon swell the ranks of arthritis sufferers. More than half of people with arthritis are diagnosed before age 65, and arthritis is the second leading cause of U.S. work disability after heart disease. Each year, approximately 39 million physician visits, 500,000 hospitalizations, and $86.2 billion in economic consequences can be attributed to arthritis.

The causes of arthritis are diverse and include joint injury, overuse, and infections as well as congenital disorders. Typically, arthritis produces nociceptive pain—a dull aching in affected joints. However, arthritis can also trigger neuropathic pain in the form of sharp pains, tingling, and numbness.

Osteoarthritis. Osteoarthritis is the most common type of arthritis. Also known as *degenerative joint disease,* it develops gradually after age 40 in the hips, knees, lower back, hands, and neck (cervical spine). Why it develops is not understood, but risks are greater in individuals who have a family history of osteoarthritis, are overweight or sedentary, have fractured or overused a joint, or have sustained a nerve injury.

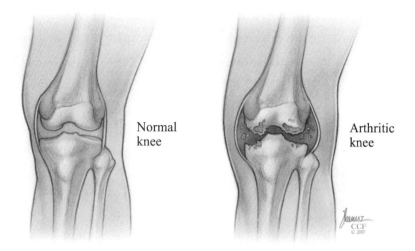

Normal knee

Arthritic knee

The figure on the right shows loss of cartilage (bearing surface) resulting from arthritic inflammation.

Osteoarthritis erodes the cartilage that lines and serves as a shock absorber for the joints. The loss of that cartilage cushion produces direct and painful bone-on-bone contact. The pain can be severe, to the point where the patient cannot bear weight.

Rheumatoid Arthritis. Rheumatoid arthritis is most common among women between 30 and 50 years of age, but it affects children as well. Caused by an abnormal immune-system response, rheumatoid arthritis triggers inflammation that swells the linings of numerous small joints in the

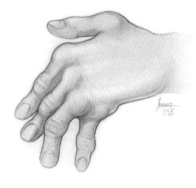

Rheumatoid arthritis

hands, feet, or cervical spine (in the neck). Typically, these joints become tender, red, and swollen during flare-ups, when fluid collects within the joint. The end result is usually joint deformity and limited movement.

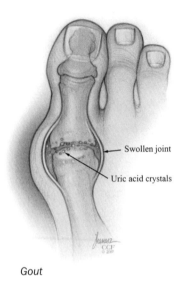

Swollen joint

Uric acid crystals

Gout

Gout. Gout is not just the affliction that plagued rich noblemen in the past. It is a form of arthritis that is alive and well today, still favoring men more than women. Caused by impaired processing of uric acid in the body, gout produces intense attacks of pain, redness, warmth, and swelling in certain joints, most notably the big toe.

Fibromyalgia. Fibromyalgia is an arthritis-related syndrome that produces severe pain in muscles, tendons, and ligaments throughout the body. (It is described in greater detail on page 60.)

Lupus. Lupus or systemic lupus erythematosus (SLE) is a chronic and painful disease that causes problems throughout the body as the immune system mistakenly targets normal connective tissue in joints, muscles, heart, lungs, skin, kidneys, and the nervous system. The cause of the chronic and painful syndrome is unknown, but lupus is eight to ten times more common in women, striking them during the childbearing years. African American women are at greatest risk.

Headache

Sonia, 30, has suffered from migraines since she was 15, just as her mother did. If she misses a meal or a good night's sleep, she has to take refuge in a darkened bedroom for an entire day to "sleep it off."

Headaches are defined as any pain around the head, behind the eyes, or between the neck and the back of the head. First described by the ancient Babylonians and Sumerians, headaches are the most common pain symptom in the United States. Each year, American rack up 8 million visits to the doctor because of headaches.

Approximately 45 million of us report chronic headaches, and half of us consider them to be severe or disabling, according to the American Pain Foundation. During a yearlong survey by the National Pain Foundation (*www.painconnection. org*), headaches were found to last:

- 1–5 days for 40 percent of respondents
- 6–10 days for 25 percent of respondents
- 11–30 days for 16 percent of respondents
- 31–100 days for 8 percent of respondents
- More than 100 days for 5 percent of respondents

The three main headache disorders are migraine, cluster, and tension headaches.

Migraines. Migraine headaches affect 25 to 30 million Americans between the ages of 15 and 55. They are a huge problem for our society. Each year, migraines are responsible for a staggering 157 million lost days of work, at a cost of $17 billion.

Women are three times as likely as men to develop these vascular headaches, which are triggered by the release of chemicals from the trigeminal nerve in the face. The chemicals irritate and swell blood vessels that wrap around the brain. The result is typically moderate to intense pulsating or throbbing pain on one side of the head—typically around the eye or temple. Migraines last 4 to 72 hours and sometimes even longer.

The clearest indications of a migraine are the presence of nausea or vomiting, extreme sensitivity to light and sound, and in 20 percent of migraine sufferers, an *aura*. Auras may involve a disturbance in vision, tingling sensations, or difficulty speaking, and they herald the onset of migraine within 20 minutes to an hour.

Cluster Headaches. Most often striking men over age 40, cluster headaches earn their name because they cluster over periods of weeks or months, then disappear for months or years at a time. These vascular headaches arise from swollen, pulsating blood vessels on one side of the head. Burning, piercing pain usually starts behind one eye and spreads across that side of the face, causing flushing, tearing, and sweating. Cluster headaches typically attack with little warning, sometimes more than once a day in the same area. Pain may last from minutes to hours and is severe enough to awaken a person from sleep, serving as an unwelcome alarm clock.

Tension Headaches. Tension headaches are the most common type of headache, with nine out of ten American adults having experienced them. Also called muscle-contraction headaches, they arise from the tightening of muscles in the scalp and neck in reaction to stress or anxiety, holding the head in one position for prolonged periods (while at the computer, for example), and other factors, including eyestrain, fatigue, and excessive caffeine or nicotine intake. Tension headaches usually produce mild to moderate pain that feels like a vise gripping the head or like dull pressure all over. The pain is mainly felt in the scalp, temples, or back of the neck.

Headaches can also serve as secondary symptoms of a primary problem such as head injury, high blood pressure, brain tumor, stroke, fever, or infection. In order to determine what type of headache you have, physicians will take a careful history, asking about its onset, duration, character, location, and possible causes. They will perform a physical exam and will sometimes order laboratory work as well as testing such as a CT (computed tomography) or an MRI (magnetic resonance imaging) scan of the head to help them make their diagnosis.

Backache: A Big Pain Indeed

Larry, 32, is a truck driver who injured his back when he caught a falling crate as he was loading it onto his rig. Bonnie, 40, is a receptionist who sits at a desk all day; she injured her back bending over to reach into a file drawer. Both have missed work and can't make it through the day without pain relievers.

After the headache, back pain is the second most common form of chronic pain in America. Our backs are integral to almost everything we do, and our lower backs bear most of the burden because our bodies bend there. For that reason, low back pain is extremely common and quite disabling.

Low back pain affects more than three-quarters of all Americans at some time in their lives. In fact, low back pain is the leading cause of disability in the United States for people under age 45, according to the American Pain Foundation. There are many causes of back pain.

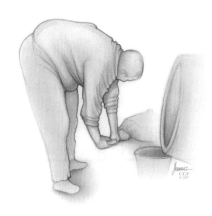

Certain occupations leave a person vulnerable to strain of the back muscles.

Back Strain. Back strain, the main cause of back pain, results from straining the muscles and ligaments that shore up the spine. It may be difficult to pinpoint exactly when back pain begins, because repeated stresses over the years build up until suddenly something just gives way. The triggering event often occurs after heavy lifting if we ignore body mechanics, or when we suddenly twist the spine—especially when we are out of shape. Sometimes the back muscles go into spasm. Most back strain resolves within several weeks with a combination of rest, exercises to recondition our protective back muscles, and training in good body mechanics.

Ruptured (Herniated) Disks. Ruptured (herniated) disks can cause the gel-like material that cushions each vertebra to bulge, pressing on the spinal cord or nerve root as we flex and extend our spines. Pain that arises from a bulging disk is typically referred along the complete pathway of the affected

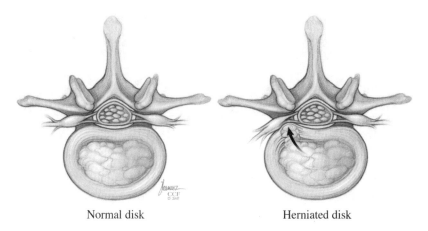

Normal disk   Herniated disk

Ruptured (herniated) disks can cause the gel-like material that cushions each vertebra to bulge, pressing on the spinal cord or nerve root.

nerve, with telltale pain reflecting its origins. For instance, pain from a ruptured disk in the cervical spine may extend over the shoulder, shoulder blade, and chest, weakening the muscles supplied by that nerve.

Sciatica. Sciatica is pain caused by a ruptured disk pressing on the sciatic nerve, which extends from the lower spine down along the back of the leg. Because pain is triggered with sideways movement of the spine, people who are afflicted with sciatica limit their movements, and their muscles further lose conditioning.

Spinal Stenosis. Spinal stenosis is a narrowing of the canal through which the spinal cord runs, as well as a narrowing of its opening(s) where nerve roots emerge. The canal can narrow because of arthritis or bony overgrowth. The result is a pinched nerve, with back and leg pain that is aggravated by walking.

Spondylosis. Spondylosis is arthritis of the intervertebral disks (which control movement of individual vertebrae in the spine), limiting flexibility. This type of arthritis causes disabling pain in the back and buttocks and behind the thighs. Spondylolisthesis often occurs in adolescents, when one vertebra slips forward over another in the spinal column. It can also occur in adults when there is a fracture or degeneration of a disk and a vertebra has slipped over another. The condition occurs in adolescents because the growth plate is not fully developed. It may resolve in a growth spurt.

Spinal Injuries. Injury to the spine and to the ligaments and muscles attached to it can be very painful. If penetrating wounds or surgery damages the peripheral nerves, chronic neuropathic pain can develop, with burning and electrical sensations distributed along the affected nerve. Repeated spine surgeries can lead to chronic pain, as can repeated episodes of acute back pain. In 28 to 40 percent of the surgeries performed to relieve nerve compression or remove bone fragments, back pain persists after the surgery. In addition, the intimate covering (arachnoid membrane) surrounding the spinal fluid may become inflamed, causing chronic pain (arachnoiditis). While surgery may be associated with arachnoiditis, it can occur after trauma, infection, or injectable substances causing chronic neuropathic pain in the back and legs with loss of sensation and, in some cases, weakness or loss of motor function. Similarly, with other chronic pain states, the failure to provide adequate pain control can lead to anxiety, stress due to wage loss, increased cost of treatment, issues with workers' compensation (if work-related), and development of psychological factors including depression.

Neuralgias: A Shock to the System

There are still other causes of chronic pain. One of these, neuralgia, produces acute spasms of sharp, burning, electric pain along the course of a nerve, with muscle weakness and sometimes sweating and temperature disturbance in the nerve region. The location of the affected nerve determines the type and location of the pain produced. Following are some common neuralgias.

Trigeminal Neuralgia. Once called *tic douloureux,* this type of neuralgia causes frequent episodes of pain arising along the trigeminal nerve in the face. The neuralgia can be caused by injury, infection, a tumor, or a metabolic disorder. This extremely debilitating disorder produces moderate to severe burning or aching pain, interrupted by brief sharp spasms. Patient may notice exquisite skin sensitivity or a dull tingling when touched. Severe shocklike pains can occur out of the blue, provoked by touching the skin of the face, chewing, or talking. Patients with trigeminal neuralgia can become extremely depressed by the frequent episodes of pain. Atypical facial pain is another form of neuralgia affecting many branches of the trigeminal nerve. A continuous aching, cramping pain involves the entire side of the face and even the neck and back of the head.

Post-herpetic Neuralgia. Commonly known as shingles, this condition involves an outbreak of fluid-filled blisters arising from nerve fibers that extend to the skin. Once you've had chickenpox, the virus that caused it (*varicella zoster*) appears to lie low in your nervous system. Later—perhaps decades later, when your immune system is weakened by age, illness, or even grief—the virus reactivates. Often, the trigeminal nerve in the face is affected. Burning, tingling, or numbness may herald the onset of shingles. This may be closely followed by fever, chills, headache, and stomachache. Several days later, painful blisters appear on a patch of flushed skin. The pain, termed *post-herpetic neuralgia,* intensifies with time and may persist for months or years. In these instances, the pain can be so agonizing that it interferes with tasks of daily living and independence, leading to depression, social isolation, and even suicidal ideation.

Occipital Neuralgia. Occipital neuralgia occurs when the occipital nerve at the back of the head is damaged or inflamed. Severe, throbbing pain develops at the back of the head and sometimes extends to involve the front of the head and eyes. With this form of neuralgia, patients complain of extreme sensitivity over the scalp.

Repetitive Motion Disorders

When the same physical actions are repeated day in and day out, the repetition takes a toll on the musculoskeletal system. Repetitive motion disorders (primarily ones that affect the wrist) are common in the workplace; in fact, upper-extremity repetitive motion disorders affect 44 of every 10,000 workers in the United States. In addition, more than half the sports-related injuries that result in visits to the doctor's office arise from the performance of the same maneuvers over and over again. Repetitive motion injuries often affect musicians, such as pianists and violinists. The most common repetitive motion disorders are tendinitis and bursitis.

Tendinitis. Tendinitis—the inflammation of the strong cord-like tissue that connects muscle to bone within the joints—leads to swelling and irritation of surrounding tissues, preventing full range of motion. Inflammation causes redness, warmth, swelling, and pain. With repeated use, chronic pain can set in. The names of the various forms of tendinitis indicate where the inflammation occurs: swimmer's shoulder, tennis elbow, jumper's knee, Achilles tendinitis, trigger finger.

Tendinitis may be complicated by nerve involvement. The median nerve, which passes from the forearm to the palm

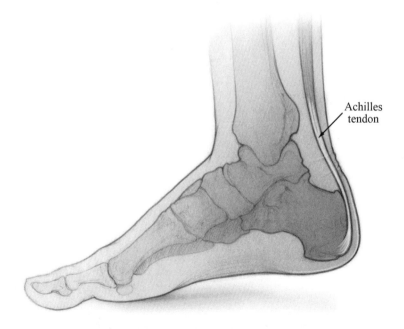

Achilles tendon

Inflammation of the Achilles tendon (shown) is an example of tendinitis.

through the carpal tunnel at the wrist, is highly susceptible to overuse injury. Involvement of the radial nerve, running along the forearm, is also susceptible to neuropathic pain in addition to musculoskeletal dysfunction. These nerve problems are responsible for highly debilitating chronic pain.

Bursitis. Bursitis is inflammation of the bursa, a small fluid-filled sac that streamlines movement by serving as a cushion between moving bones, muscles, tendons, and skin. The 150 or so bursas throughout the human body prevent friction and fraying of soft tissues and allow them to smoothly glide over bone and joints. When the normally slippery sacs swell and roughen from inflammation, movement becomes painful. Bursitis most often strikes the shoulder, elbow, hip, and knee, but can occur in other parts of the body as well.

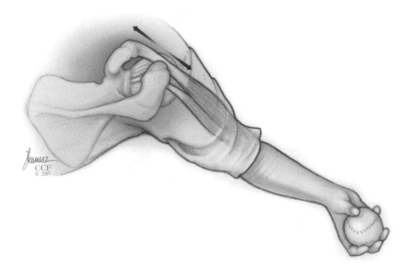

Throwing a baseball is an extreme motion that may cause inflammation of the shoulder bursa, resulting in chronic pain.

Pointed Questions

To diagnose the source of shoulder pain, your doctor will ask several questions, including:

- Does your shoulder feel comfortable when your arm is resting at your side?
- Can you reach the small of your back to tuck in your shirt with your hand?

Repeated use of the shoulder, for example by pitchers in baseball, can injure the body's most complex and vulnerable joint. The protective bursa becomes inflamed along with neighboring rotator-cuff tendons. Add tendinitis to bursitis and you have *shoulder impingement syndrome.* Friction between bones, tendons, and soft tissue causes pain with every movement. Repeated inflammation roughens and thickens bursa and tendons, which become pinched within the confined shoulder space.

Temporomandibular Joint Dysfunction. Temporomandibular joint dysfunction (TMJ) originates in the muscles around the ear that move the jaw as we chew and extends to the face, mouth, teeth, and head. It is believed to arise from incorrect positioning of jaw components due to injury, or from tension and stress that spur repeated clenching of the jaw and grinding of the teeth. In some cases, a congenital abnormality may be responsible for the dysfunction. Temporomandibular joint dysfunction can be extremely debilitating. Patients with TMJ dysfunction report clicking

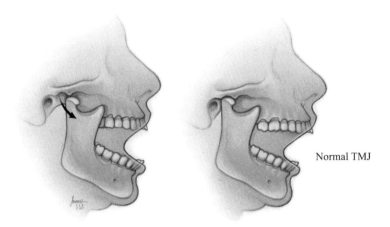

Normal TMJ

As seen in the figure on the left, exaggerated displacement of the temporomandibular joint can cause strain, ultimately leading to chronic pain.

and periodic locking of the joint, ringing in the ears, spasticity of the chewing muscles, and restrictive jaw movement, all stemming from the pain.

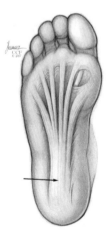

Plantar fasciitis is inflammation of the plantar fascia—a fibrous band of tissue connecting the heel bone with the bones in the forefoot.

Plantar Fasciitis. Plantar fasciitis, an extremely stubborn form of heel pain for which women are most at risk, is most severe upon stepping out of bed first thing in the morning. Overuse—the result of standing at work all day on hard surfaces, for instance, or a repetitive motion like jogging—can damage the plantar fascia, the tough tissue that connects our heel bone to the base of our toes, resulting in chronic pain.

Vascular Pain

Pain associated with the vascular system occurs in 30 million Americans. The most common form is peripheral artery disease, which stems from a buildup of fatty deposits and plaque in the arteries of the legs. When people afflicted with the buildup attempt exercises which require oxygen for energy, such as walking, their clogged blood vessels simply can't deliver oxygen to the calf muscles fast enough. Symptoms include cramping, tightness in the calf or thigh muscles, and extreme fatigue. If arterial blockage is widespread, the pain also may be present at rest. Typically, the pain is burning, constant, severe, and worse at night and when lying down.

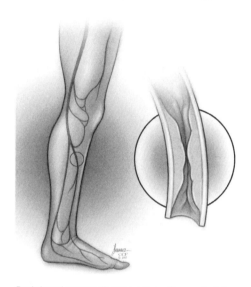

Peripheral artery disease stems from a buildup of fatty deposits and plaque in the arteries of the legs, reducing blood flow.

Deep Vein Thrombosis. When the deep veins of the legs suffer from poor circulation, a blood clot can form in the calf or thigh. Deep vein thrombosis (thrombophlebitis) causes painful swelling. Varicose veins—the enlarged, blue, crooked veins that appear on the surface of the legs—can increase susceptibility to deep vein thrombosis.

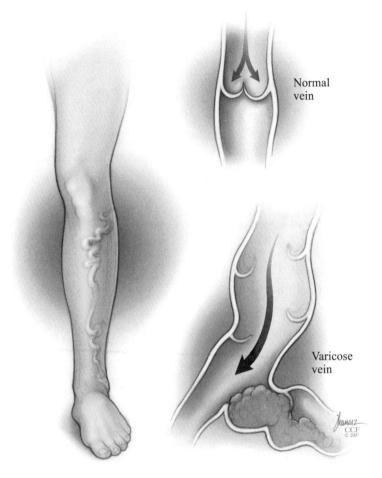

Normal
vein

Varicose
vein

Deep vein thrombosis: When the deep veins of the legs suffer from poor circulation, a blood clot can form in the calf or thigh.

Raynaud's Phenomenon. During the late 19th century, Maurice Raynaud described the constriction of small blood vessels caused by cold or an exaggerated sympathetic response. The condition occurs more frequently in women and affects the hands more often than the feet. Because its cause is unknown, it is termed *idiopathic.* Raynaud's disease as described above is associated with poor blood flow causing brief episodes of aching, throbbing, swelling, and tingling, as well as a blue tinge in the skin. Raynaud's phenomenon describes similar changes which are often a sign of connective tissue disorders, such as lupus, scleroderma, arterial occlusive diseases, trauma, and some drugs, including ergotamine.

Myofascial Pain Syndromes

The myofascia is a layer of connective tissue that envelops muscles, tendons, and ligaments. The trigger points in myofascial pain syndrome are called *jump signs* for pain. Press one of them and you'll cause pain as well as a visible twitch in the affected muscle. Persistent or spasmodic aching and tightness make sufferers restrict movement, ultimately causing muscle contractures. Myofascial pain can become debilitating because the longer that pain persists in a given muscle or group of muscles, the more likely it is to spread to adjacent muscles in the leg or trunk. Eventually, myofascial pain syndrome can cover fairly large areas of the body.

Undiagnosed and untreated myofascial pain can delay recovery from severe injuries. For example, if low back pain from a workplace injury evolves into myofascial pain syndrome, the pain can disable patients for six months or longer. Early recognition of telltale trigger points and prompt treatment are crucial to preventing long-term disability and pain.

More than one disorder results in musculoskeletal pain, or *myalgia,* but some of the most common are trauma, sports injuries, inflammatory myopathies, viral myositis, polymyalgia rheumatica, neurogenic myalgia, drug-induced myalgia, or fibromyalgia.

Fibromyalgia. The American Pain Foundation classifies fibromyalgia as one of the myofascial pain syndromes.

Fibromyalgia produces early morning stiffness and pain in muscles, ligaments, tendons, and soft tissues all over the body, as well as fatigue. It often gives rise to the question "Why am I always tired and aching?"

Fibromyalgia patients may feel bone-tired all the time, even right after waking from what should have been restorative sleep. Many characterize their pain as deep, aching, throbbing, radiating, and occasionally as burning or stabbing. The skin may become so sensitive to touch that patients will say, "It just feels like sunburn all over." For some, pain diminishes as the day wears on, only to return in the evening.

Five times more common in women than in men, fibromyalgia is usually diagnosed between ages 20 and 50. Patients often suffer from sleep disturbances, headache, numbness in the hands and feet, depression, and anxiety. Pain may be aggravated by activity, cold or damp weather, and stress.

Fibromyalgia was once considered a psychosomatic illness, but in 1990 the American College of Rheumatology recognized it as a legitimate diagnosis, based on two criteria:

- A history of widespread pain above and below the waist on both sides of the body, lasting for at least three months
- Presence of pain in at least 11 of 18 tender-point sites on the neck, shoulders, chest, rib cage, lower back, thighs, knees, arms (elbows), and buttocks

The diagnosis of fibromyalgia is complicated by its association with irritable bowel syndrome and bladder disorders, and the fact that it is a secondary complication of lupus, rheumatoid arthritis, and Lyme disease. Fibromyalgia can be distinguished from rheumatoid and other forms of arthritis because the tell-tale joint swelling and deterioration associated with arthritis are absent. In addition, the soft-tissue tender points of fibro-myalgia differ from the specific trigger points of other myofas-cial pain syndromes. These tender points in muscles send pain radiating outward and sometimes occur in isolation.

Injuries. *Consider the case of Dick, a 45-year-old sales rep who flies frequently for his job. He constantly lugs around his laptop case while he travels, and hefting the heavy bag has brought on shoulder pain that seems to be worsening. He can actually see the muscle twitching in his shoulder where it hurts.*

Acute workplace or auto injuries (bone fractures, deep bruising in a limb or trunk, or major nerve injuries) can set off myofascial pain syndrome. For example, although whiplash (hyperextension-hyperflexion) typically resolves, the impact of whiplash on joints, disks, ligaments, muscles, and nerve roots in the cervical spine can trigger myofascial pain syn-drome. Similarly, sudden overuse of muscles during weekend athletics can also invite myofascial pain, as can demanding fitness programs that involve repetitive use of certain muscles. Subtle repetitive stress injuries can also be at the root of myo-fascial pain syndrome, as with Dick's shoulder injury.

Complex Regional Pain Syndrome

Heather, 33, fractured her wrist when she fell while rollerblad-ing. The bones healed, but the pain in her wrist never let up. In fact, it spread to her entire arm, which feels as if it's constantly on fire. Heather cannot sleep or concentrate at work; her arm feels hot at times, cold at other times, and it changes color. She feels as if she's losing her mind.

Complex regional pain syndrome (CRPS) was first described during the American Civil War by Silas Weir Mitchell, a neurologist who coined the term *causalgia* to describe the intense, burning pain, glossy skin, wide temperature variations, exaggerated response to touch, and altered mental-health status of soldiers who had suffered injuries to major nerves. During World War II, anesthesiologist John Bonica observed similar symptoms of exaggerated pain response and marked disability among wounded GIs. Bonica later adopted the term *reflex sympathetic dystrophy*, or RSD, which was introduced by J. A. Evans in 1943.

Recently, a consensus panel made up of physicians and basic scientists decided the older terminology poorly described the medical syndrome and tended to determine a treatment which in many cases not only adversely affected the outcome, but also frequently led to failure of diagnosis.

The name *complex regional pain syndrome* was chosen to describe both problems, with CRPS 1 referring to reflex sympathetic dystrophy, and CRPS 2 referring to causalgia (implying major nerve injury). Both groups of patients share a history of trauma and such vulnerability to pain that simple air movement or a light touch can prompt deep, intense, burning pain at the injured site. In addition, the traumatized areas swell and develop changes in skin temperature and color. The extreme pain frequently interrupts patients' sleep.

Complex regional pain syndrome commonly develops in the limbs, but it may also appear in the knee, shoulder, head, breast, or any area of the body. From those areas, pain may spread to another extremity and eventually may involve all four extremities at once. Because of severe pain and loss of function, patients may be confined to a wheelchair or may become entirely unable to use their extremities.

Although CRPS can occur as early as age 4 and as late as age 84, most patients develop the syndrome in their late 30s or early 50s, usually as a result of trauma. But complex regional pain syndrome can develop without any history of injury. The impact of the condition on patients is devastating: Unable to work, they become understandably distressed when they learn their condition is permanent. They can become severely depressed and withdrawn. It should be noted that psychological factors do not predispose patients to CRPS. Most studies have proved that any psychological changes occur as a result, not a cause, of the condition.

Central Pain Syndrome

Most distressing to afflicted patients is chronic pain caused by damage to or dysfunction of the central nervous system (the spinal cord and brain). Central pain syndrome can be caused by stroke, multiple sclerosis, brain or spinal cord injuries, tumors, epilepsy, and Parkinson's disease. The distribution of symptoms and the effects those symptoms have on individual patients vary greatly.

Usually chronic, central pain is described as a burning sensation accompanied by tingling, pressure, and shooting or aching pain. Feelings of numbness may alternate with brief bursts of sharp pain. Beginning anywhere from soon after an injury to years after a stroke, central pain is intensified by touch, movement, emotions, and cold.

Injuries to the spinal cord, in addition to causing weakness or paralysis, may produce steady pains of a severe and burning or sharp and shooting nature. Incredible sensitivity of the skin in affected areas occurs in tandem with sensations that patients describe as a "background burning."

Pain arising in the brain is even more unbearable than pain arising in the spinal cord, because it is steady and unremitting. Central pain arising in the brain most commonly

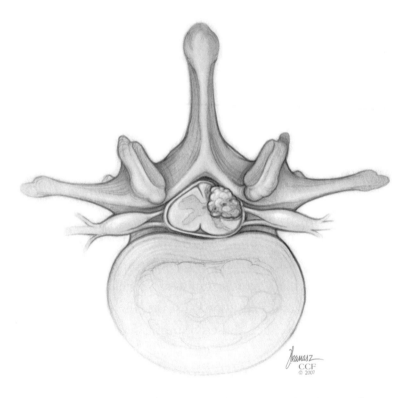

A spinal cord tumor (shown) can cause disabling pain through damage to the central nervous system.

occurs in the aftermath of a stroke. Fortunately, only 1 to 2 percent of strokes incur this challenging complication.

Phantom Pain

Phantom pain, or pain after amputation of a body part, is one of most difficult chronic pain syndromes to endure. As Bonica described, phantom pain severely tries the psychological and physical endurance of the patient as well as the therapeutic skills of the physician.

Most phantom pain develops in precisely that area of the body where the amputation took place. Patients describe it as burning, cramping, aching, bothersome, crushing, or pulling. Symptoms typically last for at least ten years, although for some more fortunate patients, they diminish within months or one year.

Many patients who experience phantom pain bounce from doctor to doctor and clinic to clinic, seeking relief that all too frequently remains elusive. They undergo repeated medical and surgical interventions in the hope that the next one will provide the cure, only to find that it, too, fails as miserably as the previous attempts.

The intensity of phantom pain varies from patient to patient. Some experience it as a mere annoyance, while in other patients the condition disrupts sleep, interferes with work, and produces a profound effect on the psyche. The mechanism of phantom pain is well understood, but the clinical means of reducing the symptoms remain poor or experimental. As with many other neuropathic pain disorders—including stroke and post-herpetic neuralgia—neural systems in the phantom pain sufferer's central nervous system become sensitized to chronic pain impulses, and ultimately, develop new pain generators that accurately reproduce pain that would ordinarily be felt in the amputated body part.

Chapter 5

Pain and Cancer

Why devote an entire chapter of our book to cancer pain? Because everyone knows someone whose life has been touched by cancer. After all, cancer is the second leading cause of death in this country after cardiovascular disease.

A diagnosis of cancer rocks a family to its roots. Patients, friends, and loved ones immediately seek out as much information as possible about it and spend endless hours speculating about its cause. In the process, they hear horror stories about cancer and its treatment.

One of the greatest worries for a cancer patient is pain. And with good reason: at least 33 percent of patients receiving treatment for cancer suffer significant pain. That proportion rises to 90 percent in patients with advanced cancer. In addition, as many as 20 percent of adult cancer patients suffer pain as a result of therapy.

It is natural for cancer patients to fear that their pain may not be adequately controlled. And their fear is well founded because, in fact, cancer pain is frequently undertreated. Compounding the problem is that cancer patients fear both side effects from and addiction to painkillers.

But the truth is that people with cancer do not need to endure pain. This message is clearly spelled out in the National Cancer Institute's (NCI) detailed *Pain Control: A Guide for People with Cancer and Their Families.* (You can find the booklet on the Web at *www.cancer.gov/cancertopics/paincontrol/allpages* as well as at several other sites.) The guide also offers tips for talking with doctors and nurses. For cancer patients, pain is a warning signal that should be reported immediately. Early determination of the source of a new symptom will alert the patient's physician (oncologist) to not only provide pain relief but also undertake treatment that may remove or minimize the impact of its root cause.

When cancer patients are free of pain, they sleep better, eat better, and actively engage in family life, friendships, and careers. The NCI asserts that cancer patients have a right to ask for pain relief—and that doing so is not a sign of weakness.

Although many medical institutions display a patient's bill of rights that includes the institution's commitment to providing optimal pain management along with cancer treatment, in reality many patients suffer unnecessarily. As a result, the World Health Organization, the American Pain Society, the Agency for Healthcare Policy and Research, the American Society of Anesthesiologists, and other organizations have issued pain-management guidelines. Physicians and health-care workers at every institution are expected to create a plan for pain management, to follow its protocols, and to seek expert consultation when necessary.

Why Is Cancer Pain Undertreated?

Cancer pain is undertreated in the United States for a number of reasons. Patients tend to avoid reporting symptoms because they fear that pain is an indication that their disease may be progressing. Some treating physicians may not prescribe adequate pain medication because they are overly concerned about narcotic abuse and legal liability. Other physicians may not be well versed in evaluating cancer pain or about contemporary pain-management techniques.

Other contributing factors include:

- A lack of national policies driving palliative care and pain relief

- A lack of awareness that most cancer pain is treatable

- A shortfall of financial resources to support appropriate pain management by adequately trained personnel

- Tension between appropriate use of prescription medication and fear of psychological dependence or drug abuse

What Causes Cancer Pain?

Cancer pain has many causes, including the tumor itself and the different avenues of treatment. Cancer pain may be nociceptive or neuropathic, and constant or sporadic (so-called *breakthrough pain*).

Nociceptive pain—pain that is dull, aching, and confined to a specific area—may stem from cancer itself, as when a tumor invades the bone and fractures it or when a tumor blocks the bowel or the urinary tract.

Neuropathic pain—pain that is constant, sharp, burning, and accompanied by electrical spasms that shoot along an affected nerve to distant sites—arises when growing tumors place pressure on nerves or the spinal cord, or when tumors secrete substances that irritate the nerves.

The cancer diagnosis process may also cause discomfort. Procedures such as biopsies (taking tissue samples to determine the type and stage of cancer) may be painful. And the mainstays of cancer treatment—radiation therapy, chemotherapy, and surgery—used alone or in combination can give rise to pain in different ways.

How Does Radiation Therapy Cause Pain?

Radiation therapy, or radiotherapy, may be the most widely used cancer treatment. Used to destroy or shrink tumors, radiotherapy can damage skin and mucous membranes, and scar nerves at the treatment site. Radiation-induced injury to the brachial plexus (the network of nerves supplying the shoulders and arms) or to the lumbosacral plexus (the nerves supplying the lower extremities) causes neuropathic pain, in the same manner as has been described in other conditions in which injured nerves may cause certain neurons in the central nervous system that are involved in the pain pathways to become sensitized. As has been described earlier, neuropathic pain is undoubtedly the most intractable, most severe, and most distressing of chronic pain conditions.

How Does Chemotherapy Cause Pain?

Chemotherapy relies on powerful drugs that are toxic to cancers to shrink some early tumors or kill cancer cells that have spread throughout the body. But these poisonous agents can also be toxic to nerves, producing peripheral neuropathy, or burning pain in the hands and feet. This form of neuropathic pain can occur in conjunction with nociceptive pain in the mouth and throat, caused by the mouth sores that frequently accompany chemotherapy. Further complications include headaches, stomachaches, and painful infections that arise after chemotherapy destroys protective cells in a patient's immune system. And, as in Nancy's case, hardware used to make the delivery of the chemotherapy easier may also cause discomfort and pain, especially if the site where the hardware is installed becomes infected.

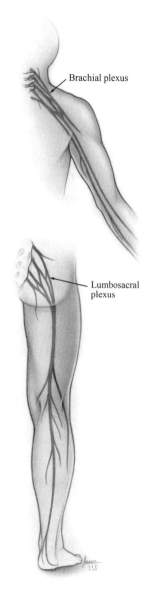

Brachial plexus

Lumbosacral plexus

Radiation-induced injury to the brachial plexus, the network of nerves supplying the shoulder and arm (top), or to the lumbosacral plexus, the nerves supplying the lower extremities (bottom), causes neuropathic pain.

Nancy

Nancy was 57 when she noticed a feeling of fullness in her abdomen. She sought help from her doctors, who suspected ovarian cancer. Nancy's doctors elected to perform a total hysterectomy to remove what they believed to be a tumor. During the course of the surgery, however, they found that the sensations Nancy was experiencing arose from cancer in the lymph nodes in her abdomen. The diagnosis: non-Hodgkin's lymphoma.

Fairly active and in relatively good health, Nancy recovered from the major surgery uneventfully. Chemotherapy was prescribed, and she struggled a bit to gain weight, as her oncologists advised, to better manage her chemotherapy. To simplify delivery of the chemotherapy drugs, the doctors installed a temporary port in Nancy's arm. Shortly after her first session, Nancy went out shopping with her daughters but began to feel ill during their excursion. The arm into which the port had been implanted began to swell at an alarming rate. The tissue around the port looked red and felt warm, and Nancy developed a fever.

A real trooper when it came to pain, Nancy was reluctant to go to the hospital. But her daughters observed that she was rapidly heading downhill as her pain increased. They took her to the emergency room of a busy hospital in the city, where Nancy had to sit in the waiting room for several hours. Finally, her daughters made clear the gravity of her situation, and the physicians gave Nancy a dose of Dilaudid (hydromorphone hydrochloride). At that point, the powerful narcotic proved to be the only medication that could touch her pain.

Euphoric at finding relief from the dizzying pain, Nancy worried that she could become dependent on the narcotic. But she was reassured that addiction or dependence is not a concern when a strong narcotic is given in response to severe pain. The cause of Nancy's pain was finally identified when Nancy was diagnosed with a staph infection. She spent a week in the hospital to recover from the infection, which delayed her chemotherapy. Nancy's spirits sank as her hair began falling out in clumps.

In response to Nancy's depression, her family convinced the doctors that she would recover faster emotionally and physically if she could recuperate at home. The doctors agreed, and once her infection was under control, Nancy was discharged.

This case highlights the competition between the extreme emotional and psychological issues associated with a life-threatening illness and the natural desire and preference to be home rather than in an institution. Pitted against these conflicting desires is the physician's goal to provide the best possible medical care. While they witnessed the interplay between their mother and her medical needs, Nancy's daughters had had their first experience in advocating on behalf of a loved one in pain.

How Does Cancer Surgery Cause Pain?

Cancer surgery is performed less often today than it was in the past, but it may be deployed to relieve pain by clearing bowel obstructions or removing a bony tumor that is pinching the spinal cord. But the surgery itself can cause both nociceptive and neuropathic pain. For example, when a lung cancer is removed, injury to the intercostal (chest) nerves can give rise to neuropathic pain and skin hypersensitivity around the surgical scar. Removal of cancerous lymph nodes in the neck may refer pain along nerves to the head, shoulder, jaw, ear, or even the upper chest.

Postsurgical phantom pain is an insidious type of neuropathic pain. After breast removal, for example, mastectomy patients often develop sensations of burning, numbness, and tightening along the chest wall, armpit, and arm. Shoulder movement heightens the extreme sensitivity of skin around the incision, so the mastectomy patient may opt to hold her shoulder still to avoid rubbing against a sensitive area. The lack of motion may, in turn, lead to the development of adhesive capulitis, commonly called frozen shoulder, a very painful condition that will compound the phantom the patient is already enduring.

Addressing Psychological Factors

As was true in Nancy's experience, pain influences the psychological state of most cancer patients. About 45 percent of patients suffering from cancer pain develop psychological problems such as anxiety, depression, and even delirium. It's important to identify these conditions early so they, too, can be managed.

Managing behavioral problems is as critical to cancer treatment as is managing pain and other symptoms. Fear of death, suffering, deformity, financial difficulties, and loneliness actually increase our perception of pain. If untreated,

When You Need a Pain Specialist

The National Cancer Institute recommends that families seek out a pain specialist if the treating physician cannot provide adequate pain control. To locate a specialist, families can contact their local cancer center, hospice, or the oncology department at a nearby medical center. The NCI's Cancer Information Service (on the Web at *http://cis.nci.nih.gov*) and the American Cancer Society (*www.cancer.org*) are other potential resources for pain-management facilities, pain specialists, and pain clinics or programs in your area.

depression and withdrawal will harm relationships with loved ones, and as has been shown in many studies, may not only weaken a patient's will to live but can physically shorten his or her life.

Community-education programs aimed at increasing the understanding of cancer pain have had mixed success. Nevertheless, studies demonstrate that when patients understand more about what causes their pain, the intensity of painful symptoms is reduced by as much as 30 percent.

The best approach to cancer-pain management is interdisciplinary, requiring collaboration among the primary-care physician, oncologist, radiologist, pain specialist, psychologist or therapist, nurses, social workers, and others. Changing the patient's perception of pain through the use of pain medications, antidepressants, anxiety medications, and therapy is a key component of cancer treatment—and the right team can make this effort more successful.

Tackling Cancer Pain with Analgesics

The effective management of cancer pain begins with analgesics. In 1996, the World Health Organization developed a set of guidelines, called the "analgesic letter," to advise healthcare professionals about the most appropriate medications for pain relief. Recommended first are non-narcotics such as aspirin and acetaminophen, together with laxatives, antianxiety medications, antidepressants, and similar drugs. Nonsteroidal anti-inflammatory (NSAID) drugs are also helpful in relieving cancer pain.

The more severe the pain, the more likely it is that narcotics such as Dilaudid (hydromorphone hydrochloride), OxyContin (oxycodone), morphine, and methadone will be required. Many of these agents are available in sustained-release forms that are more acceptable to patients who may need to take medications only once or at most three times a day. In addition, short-acting medications can be prescribed for episodes of *breakthrough pain,* when discomfort increases quite suddenly. The short-acting medications provide a bridge of protection from the pain that can arise between doses of sustained-release medicine.

What if Medication Doesn't Mediate My Cancer Pain?

Sometimes medications are not effective in relieving cancer pain. Fortunately, in these cases cancer pain can be controlled with anesthetic techniques to intercept pain impulses before they reach the central nervous system. These techniques include local anesthetic blocks, infusion pumps, and neuro-modulation of pain impulses. Local anesthetic procedures can block specific nerve pathways serving the region where the pain originates. Most local nerve blocks provide rapid relief of symptoms in the affected areas and are used for diagnosis and, in some cases, treatment. Sometimes merely interrupting a source of pain may have long-lasting effects.

• • • *Fast Fact* • • •

Neuromodulation, a recently introduced term applies to the non-destructive modulation of the nervous system. One application is spinal cord stimulation, which delivers pulsed electrical energy to the spinal cord to interrupt the transmission of pain messages to the brain. Pain physicians use neuromodulation to treat cancer pain and other types of chronic pain.

• • •

A small catheter inserted under the skin or into the space around the spinal cord can provide longer-lasting relief through continuous delivery of local anesthetics, narcotics, or other pain relievers. If a trial catheter infusion of medication is successful, sometimes doctors will implant a programmable pump in a pocket just beneath the skin. This allows for delivery of appropriate amounts of medications over a long period of time. The pump reservoirs can be conveniently refilled through the skin.

In other cases, catheters are connected to external infusion pumps. Infusion pumps may serve a number of purposes

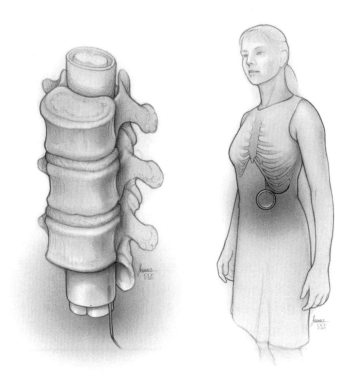

If a trial catheter infusion of medication is successful, a programmable pump may be implanted in a pocket just beneath the skin.

besides pain management: delivery of antibiotics, hydration therapy, and nutrition therapy, if necessary. Home infusion also allows for the extension of hospital services to the home environment. Such systems are tended by home-care nurses who refill the infusion system on a scheduled basis and can provide outstanding pain control not achievable by oral or intramuscular injections.

The advantage of these techniques is the dramatic reduction of drug-related side effects. Because the medicines follow a much more direct route to the pain pathways, the doses involved are just a fraction of the doses required orally. Thus, patients can avoid many of the side effects associated with large doses of narcotics such as morphine or Dilaudid. For patients' relatives, these interventions make the difference between seeing a loved one who is confused and barely awake and seeing one who is fully alert.

Quality of Life

As cancer treatments have become more successful, patients are living dramatically longer lives. Life expectancy has a significant bearing on how a patient's cancer pain is managed. When life expectancy is short, most patients who have responded well to an external infusion system can go home. Home-care services provide support for patients who are equipped with external pumps or implanted pumps that require medication refills, so patients can enjoy their home environment and be near loved ones.

Because cancer growth is so variable, symptom management may extend from a few weeks to years. Pain relief should provide the utmost comfort and the fewest side effects. Foremost among end-of-life issues is the quality of the patient's life. An aggressive approach to treating cancer may be supplanted by the need to minimize the side effects that attend cancer treatment and pain management. The goals of health-care providers are to relieve cancer symptoms as much as possible, to provide psychological support, and to enlist the help of relatives. Obviously, when life is short, pain relief is a priority. When possible, pain should be managed in a palliative care (also called *comfort care*) mode either in a hospice or, ideally, at home.

Messages from the National Cancer Institute

- Cancer patients should not try to grit their teeth and make their way unaided through pain. Untreated pain can worsen the pain, require larger doses of pain medicine, and delay cancer treatment.
- Despite the hype about prescription narcotic abuse, people who take pain relievers to alleviate cancer pain rarely become addicted.
- Narcotic and opioid doses are closely monitored by health-care providers; they may cause drowsiness, but they won't make cancer patients "high." Drowsiness is viewed as a beneficial side effect, because the sleep that follows has a therapeutic effect.
- Cancer patients whose pain is poorly managed feel tired, depressed, angry, worried, lonesome, and distressed.
- Cancer patients whose pain is well managed enjoy improvement in mood, physical activity, sociability, appetite, sleep, and sexual intimacy.
- Patients should always ask, "What other steps can I take to manage my pain?"

Cancer Pain in Children

Tackling cancer pain in children can be particularly challenging for health-care providers. To appropriately treat children's pain, physicians must be able to "speak their language." For example, children may use metaphors to describe their pain, likening severe pain to the roaring of a lion, for instance. As

Different Approaches to Treating Cancer

Psychological Approaches
- Understanding
- Cognitive behavioral
- Companionship therapies

Common Therapeutic Interventions
- Radiation therapy
- Chemotherapy
- Hormone therapy
- Surgery

Pain-Relieving Medications
- Analgesics (painkillers)
- Anxiety-relieving drugs
- Antidepressants
- Neuroleptics (antiseizure medicine)

Interruption of the Pain Pathway
- Local anesthetics
- Neurosurgery
- Infusion pumps

Modifying Daily Activities and Immobilization
- Rest
- Plastic splints or slings
- Cervical collar or corset

you'll read in chapter 7, the FACES scale, which uses universal facial expressions to convey and correspond to pain levels, and similar tools can help children describe their pain with words.

Cultural and gender differences may also influence a child's description of the severity of the pain. For example, in Asian cultures, the emphasis on self-control and obedience may discourage children from expressing pain. Pain specialists have also noted that girls from Asian and Arab cultures tend to use emotional terms, such as *sad* or *embarrassed,* to describe their pain, while their male counterparts use more aggressive terms, such as *angry* or *mad.*

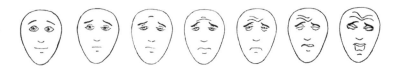

When young patients have difficulty describing pain, artistic and creative expression through maps or drawings (as shown above) can help them show what they're feeling and where it hurts. Older children may log the frequency and intensity of their pain in pain diaries.

We'll spend more time discussing the issues particular to children in pain in chapter 7.

Chapter 6

Controlling Your Pain

P ain is an abstract concept that can be defined only by the sufferer. Perhaps that is why pain management remains largely misunderstood today by physicians and health-care workers. Complicating matters is the fact that pain treatment is an imperfect science, often relying on trial and error.

The concept of multidisciplinary pain management is rooted in the fact that people are different, that they experience pain differently, that pain has different causes and produces different symptoms, and that a number of systems of the body may be involved.

The state of chronic pain itself can trigger depression, physical deconditioning, social isolation, and problems at work. The goal of any pain-treatment program is improved quality of life, but achieving that goal means addressing the medical, psychological, environmental, occupational, and social facets of life. This is a daunting task for any single physician or health-care provider.

A Coordinated Effort

A multidisciplinary team—typically consisting of a pain specialist, psychologist, psychiatrist, physical and occupational therapists, and social workers—can address treatment issues at the same time and in a coordinated fashion. Because chronic pain may be a lifelong condition, multidisciplinary pain clinics across the country emphasize coping skills, physical rehabilitation, and behavioral management.

Interestingly, many studies demonstrate that patients who complete a multidisciplinary pain-treatment program reduce or even eliminate their need for narcotic pain relievers. However, few patients actually seek out this multifaceted approach to pain management. Most focus solely on their medical needs. But rehabilitation and pain treatment go hand in hand, whether a patient is disabled by a back injury sustained at work, a sports injury, or cancer.

Pain associated with fibromyalgia serves as a good example of chronic pain that benefits from team treatment. Physical therapists help afflicted patients strengthen and increase flexibility in sore, unused muscles through exercises undertaken on land or in a pool. Psychologists offer behavioral therapy to tackle underlying depression, and psychiatrists may prescribe antidepressants that help to reestablish effective sleep patterns. Anesthesiologists can prescribe analgesics that show promise in reducing pain from fibromyalgia. The patient's primary doctor and rheumatologist are also part of this team, as they may be most familiar with the general medical state of the patient or are currently managing a rheumatological condition.

Consider Penny, a woman diagnosed with fibromyalgia who, decades ago, had given up on her life. With a proper pain management program, she now enjoys a relatively normal life.

Penny

Shortly after giving birth to her second child 32 years ago, Penny began to experience headaches. Their onset was gradual. But eventually, the headaches grew in frequency and intensity until they controlled her life.

Penny consulted doctors in her hometown in an effort to diagnose and treat her aching head and the sore neck and arm pain that accompanied it, but she never received a concrete explanation for her condition. The doctors always ran tests to try to determine the source of her pain, but the tests always came back normal.

Eventually, Penny was diagnosed with fibromyalgia, one of the diagnoses given in the past to women with unexplained symptoms. The unspoken implication was that her pain wasn't real—that she was imagining it. Penny decided to seek the opinion of a Cleveland Clinic rheumatologist.

"A big part of me wanted to give up. Any movement hurt, and I was really nonfunctional in every sense of the word. The pain was extreme. I couldn't take care of my children, my husband, my home, or myself," Penny recalls. "I agreed to go to the clinic thinking that I would

fail and prove to my husband and children that they should leave me."

To her surprise, the rheumatologist confirmed her diagnosis of fibromyalgia and told her that Cleveland Clinic had a pain specialist who could help her. Penny was skeptical, but she decided to meet with the head of the Section of Chronic Pain Rehabilitation in the Department of Psychiatry and Psychology.

On Halloween in 1979, Penny entered the intensive inpatient Chronic Pain Rehabilitation Program. Today, the program is part of the Section of Pain Medicine in the Neurological Institute. "It was the scariest experience of my life," she recalls. "The doctor said that he could help me, but I would have to be an active participant." At the time, Penny didn't know what that commitment was going to mean.

Though she arrived believing that she would fail, Penny did nothing of the kind. "There must have been some little spark buried very deep inside me that was ignited when the doctor said, 'I can help you,' when he believed that I was in pain. This form of validation was so important to the ultimate success of my treatment."

The physical part of the program was extremely challenging and grew more difficult before it got easier. Because weight-bearing and aerobic exercises improve flexibility and reduce pain in fibromyalgia, Penny found herself in a program that demanded that she remain active from morning to night.

"I couldn't hold a cup of coffee and I was being asked to lift a ten-pound weight," Penny says. Yet she listened

and absorbed everything she was told. Halfway into the program, she started feeling better physically.

Getting through an intensive multidisciplinary rehabilitation program demands more than gaining control over physical pain. Learning to manage the emotional aspects of pain takes much longer. That is why the program requires participants to look within in order to regain control of their lives.

"It was very empowering to explore who I was and how I dealt with or didn't deal with pain," says Penny. "I entered the clinic as a nonfunctioning patient whose sole identity was pain. I left seven weeks later as a real person."

What to Expect from a Pain Management Program

A good multidisciplinary program will:

- Identify and treat unresolved medical issues

- Eliminate inappropriate medications

- Identify and prescribe optimal medications

- Improve aerobic conditioning, endurance, strength, and flexibility

- Eliminate excessive guarding behaviors that interfere with normal activities

- Improve coping skills and psychological well-being

- Alleviate depression

- Assess patient resources and identify vocational and recreational opportunities

- Educate patients about pain, anatomy, physiology, and psychology, and teach them how to distinguish between *hurt* and *harm*

- Educate patients about prudent use of health-care resources

- Assist patients in establishing realistic goals and maintaining treatment gains

Getting Started: Physical and Occupational Therapy

One of the first steps toward managing chronic pain involves physical therapy. Physical therapy includes exercises that improve range of motion, strength, flexibility, and endurance, along with body mechanics. Low-impact exercises, such as walking, swimming, using elliptical trainers and recumbent bikes at the gym, and yoga, can ease pain in arthritic knees and hips. Exercise therapy gives patients with complex regional pain syndrome the best chance to achieve a respite from their condition. Patients with myofascial pain syndrome can use stretching exercises to reestablish function and movement in an affected muscle.

Occupational therapists improve a patient's capacity for self-care, work, and leisure activities. Becoming more independent, taking up hobbies, and getting vocational counseling all help people in pain feel more productive and engaged.

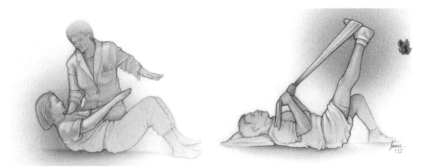

Physical therapy teaches patients exercises they can perform at home to redevelop and maintain optimal function.

All chronic pain begins as acute pain, but a vast majority of functional impairment is preventable. As the Cleveland Clinic specialist who treated Penny advised: "Keep moving, keep living, and if you're in pain, at least try to keep your life full. If your life is empty, pain will certainly fill it up." (For exercise diagrams, see Appendix 4.)

Behavioral Therapy

In the 1960s, psychologist Wilber E. Fordyce, PhD, pioneered the behavioral approach to pain at the University of Washington, which complemented the medical approach developed by his colleague John Bonica. As we saw in Penny's case, incorporating clinical psychology in a multidisciplinary rehabilitation environment adds powerfully effective tools to a patient's effort to alleviate chronic pain.

Fordyce stressed the need for a contract between patient and health-care provider, to describe the shared responsibility of managing a patient's pain. In other words, recognizing that although chronic pain often cannot be cured, pain special-ists will do their utmost to minimize symptoms and improve function. Patients, in turn, although not to be left to fend off overwhelming pain in isolation, must commit to making their pain manageable—to somehow make peace with pain.

Patients also must be encouraged to use the painful part of the body to counteract a guarding mind-set, Fordyce believed. In other words, if you injure your knee, you'll protect it ini-tially by limping. But the idea that using your knee will be too painful might take hold in your mind, and guarding the knee could become a habit. After a while, you no longer need to protect your knee, but you become stiff and your muscles lose their conditioning, worsening the problem. To resolve the problem, you must begin to use your knee and strengthen the muscles around it.

Fordyce also advanced the idea that pain itself can be a learned behavior. In other words, the presence of pain for prolonged periods can reinforce certain behaviors. Individuals who attract attention because of their pain might continue to complain of symptoms to maintain the interest and concern of others. Supporting Fordyce's findings is the documented fact that people who are involved in litigation or are receiving financial compensation because of chronic pain do not fare as well in rehabilitation.

Our relationships can also be affected by learned pain behaviors. A typical circumstance involves *learned helpless-ness,* an infantile or dependent way of behaving when others constantly care for us. Clearly, if we've been sick for the last 20 years of our lives, our relationships will change dramati-cally. It is in these cases that health-care professionals encoun-ter family role reversals, such as a 12-year-old taking care of a

40-year-old. Many of the therapy hours included in pain programs are aimed at putting those relationships back in order.

So My Pain Isn't All in My Head, but Can My Head Affect What I'm Experiencing?

It's important for you to understand that you are not imagining your pain—it is real, you are not weak, and you do not have to suffer. That said, however, chronic pain has such an immense impact on the person suffering its effects that it dramatically magnifies any preexisting psychological disorders. For example, anger, sadness, anxiety, or other stress is certain to amplify the pain level exponentially in a manner similar to cranking up the volume on a HiFi system until the sound is distorted.

Learning about *psychogenic pain,* or pain that stems from the psyche, empowers patients. An educated patient is much better equipped to cope with pain symptoms. Understanding the causes and effects of pain, and the difference between suffering and actual harm, provides reassurance that reduces anxiety and depression, improving the person's experience with pain.

Many patients have to accept that they will live with a certain amount of pain. The idea of accepting pain may seem paradoxical because it appears to be giving up or surrendering. But learning to put pain in the background can lead to productive and even joyous living.

The only place we can really suffer is in our heads. Psychological constructs feed on the physical effects and vice versa. In chronic pain, while psychological aspects may dominate, it matters little which of these comes first, as the combined impact is the same. More important is the assurance that help is available in the form of many trained health professionals who have an understanding and the tools by which these symptoms can be modified or even reversed. It may take many different interventions to address a multitude of symptoms. For example, depression, a significant component of chronic pain, cannot be reduced by yoga alone, but yoga may be integral in the management regime that is employed to deal with it and the main source—chronic pain.

Medication

Using over-the-counter analgesics such as Tylenol or Aleve and avoiding pain triggers such as caffeine and alcohol may be enough to keep chronic headaches at bay. But many other medications—local anesthetic techniques and physical interventions besides analgesics—are used to treat head pain.

Sumatriptan. When migraines strike, sumatriptan medications such as Imitrex counter blood-vessel constriction, sensitivity to light, and nausea. In addition, medications designed for entirely different purposes can halt pain in its tracks, and they can work in concert with analgesics.

Calcium Channel Blockers. Calcium channel blockers such as verapamil were developed to manage chest pain from heart disease and high blood pressure, but they are also effective in the treatment of migraine and cluster headaches.

Pain Applications for Antiseizure and Epilepsy Medications. Medications developed to treat epilepsy such as topiramate or valproate help prevent migraine and cluster headaches, while the antiseizure drug gabapentin (Neurontin) is used for different types of neuropathic pain. Carbamazepine (Tegretol) is especially helpful in trigeminal neuralgia (severe, intermittent facial pain), and pregabalin (Lyrica) helps provide symptom relief in fibromyalgia.

Antidepressants. Antidepressants such as amitriptyline (Elavil) and bupropion (Wellbutrin) can suppress the stubborn pain of peripheral neuropathy or shingles. They interfere with the pain pathway by trapping serotonin (a pain-blocking brain chemical) at the spinal cord to prolong pain relief. The sedative properties of antidepressants make them ideal for bedtime use to reestablish broken sleep patterns when pain causes fitful sleep. A good night's rest elevates our pain threshold and reduces stress and our need for analgesics.

Oral Muscle Relaxants. Oral muscle relaxants act on the central nervous system to relax the entire body and combat muscle (myofascial) pain in the legs, arms, back, or neck. The use of muscle relaxants such as tizanidine (Zanaflex) for a month in combination with regular physical or occupational therapy can reduce both pain from muscle spasms and the need for narcotics.

Does It Matter How I Take the Medication?

Yes. Sometimes the correct drug is less effective because of how or when it was delivered. Releasing a drug either more slowly or much more quickly into the body can manage symptoms more effectively.

PAIN SEVERITY	ANALGESIC TYPES	EXAMPLES
Mild (pain score: 1–3)	• oral acetaminophen	• Tylenol (acetaminophen)
	• oral nonsteroidal anti-inflammatory agents	• ibuprofen (Motrin, Advil); naproxen (NSAIDs: Aleve, Naprosyn)
Moderate (pain score: 4–6)	• intravenous (IV) NSAIDs	• ketorolac (Toradol)
	• oral acetaminophen opioid combinations	• Tylenol with codeine no. 3
Severe (pain score: 7–10)	• intravenous (IV) or epidural opioids (narcotics)	• morphine, hydromorphone (Dilaudid), fentanyl, oxycodone

For example, patients in severe chronic pain fare better with slow-release medications—particularly narcotics—because they need to be taken only at specific times each day, at intervals of 8, 12, or 24 hours. If pain spikes during a breakthrough episode, a quick-acting pain medication can be added to the mix. Fast-acting pain medications can also halt pain at its onset.

In addition, some medication is adequately absorbed by mouth (orally). Other medications are more effective when injected through the skin (transdermally), into a vein (intravenously), into a muscle (intramuscularly), or into the space surrounding the spinal cord (epidurally).

The chart above shows examples of several analgesics and the different ways they can be delivered in response to varying pain levels.

Spinal Drug-Delivery Systems. For unrelenting pain, spinal drug-delivery systems are used to infuse opiates, local anesthetics, and other medications continuously into the spine. They require an initial hospitalization so a small catheter can be inserted into the epidural space inside the spine (see the illustration on page 78). Once the catheter is in place, testing will determine the correct medications and their proper concentration for use on an outpatient basis.

When the desired level of pain relief is achieved, an external infusion pump may be used for several weeks or months. For unlimited use, a programmable, refillable pump can be implanted beneath the skin in the abdomen. These ambulatory infusion pumps allow patients to be mobile while simultaneously receiving a continuous infusion of pain medication. The pumps are easily refilled at intervals through the skin.

Do Narcotics Have Many Negative Side Effects?

Many narcotics can bring about side effects, such as constipation, nausea and vomiting, confusion, or sedation, but they are very useful in treating pain. Side effects, while uncomfortable, should not necessarily prompt you or your doctor to discontinue the use of narcotics.

Proper treatment with opioids, or narcotics derived from opium, means managing a patient's side effects. The addition of laxatives and antiemetics (medications that quell nausea) will offset side effects, and antidepressants can work in synergy with opiates to enhance their effectiveness. Then narcotic doses can be lowered.

Will I Become Dependent on Narcotics if I Take Them to Treat My Pain?

Opioids can create both physical and psychological dependence, so their use must be closely monitored. It is often true that patients who take opioids for chronic pain are not aware when they have become tolerant of prescription narcotics. Determining which factor or combination of factors has reduced the overall effectiveness of their medications can be difficult, if not impossible.

There are four reasons that increasingly strong doses of opiates may be needed:

- With time, the sites within the nervous system where the narcotic acts to relieve pain may require more drug to achieve the same effect.
- The patient may develop a psychological dependence on the drug for pain relief.
- The patient's metabolism may speed up, reducing the amount of drug available for therapeutic effect.
- There may be a real increase in actual pain.

Many patients fear becoming dependent on narcotics—however, as illustrated in several of the case studies in this book, a patient's reluctance to take narcotics often leads to worsening and unnecessary pain. A good doctor will assure you that some form of painkiller is absolutely necessary if you are suffering from severe chronic pain. Without it, you cannot perform the exercise therapy you need to regain function in the part of your body that is disabled.

Furthermore, these drugs should be given sooner, rather than later, to achieve the best effect. Do not delay taking narcotics if your doctor or pain specialist has recommended them to you. You must be able to trust your physician to manage your medication—if you do not, the appropriate action is to find a new doctor you *can* trust, not to avoid taking necessary medicine.

Nerve Blocks

Standing shoulder-to-shoulder with exercise, behavioral therapy, and medications in the management of chronic pain are nerve blocks. They are another tool in our pain-management arsenal, providing a respite from pain so rehabilitation can proceed. Most nerve blocks are not painful and provide rapid relief of symptoms in affected areas.

Anesthesiologists use nerve blocks for diagnosis, to identify exactly where the pain is coming from by isolating its source. We also use nerve blocks for treatment to prevent pain signals from transmitting along the body's nerve pathways to the brain.

At many places in the body, local anesthetics (numbing agents) can be injected near a painful nerve or group of nerves (called a *ganglion* or *plexus*), to interrupt the pain pathway for extended periods.

A facet joint block, injected into the tiny joints at the back of the spine, can stop pain signals from traveling up to your neck or down to your lower back. In conditions such as complex regional pain (also known as *reflex sympathetic dystrophy syndrome*) affecting the legs or feet, a lumbar sympathetic block can interfere with pain signals and sometimes stop the pain completely.

When the face, arms, or hands are affected by Complex Regional Pain syndrome, shingles, or phantom pain, a stellate ganglion block of nerves in the neck area can decrease pain and increase circulation.

Blocking a group of abdominal nerves known as the celiac plexus reduces pain in the upper abdomen from pancreatic and other cancers. And injections of local anesthetics between the ribs (intercostal blocks) combat chest pain arising from shingles or a surgical incision. These and many other nerve blocks are used to address painful symptoms in other parts of the body.

Sometimes small amounts of steroids can be injected with local anesthetics to reduce pain and inflammation at muscle trigger points to treat myofascial pain syndrome. This combination also helps physicians tackle pain and inflammation from nerve-entrapment syndromes in the shoulders, hands, or feet.

Is Anesthesia Used to Block Nerves?

Local anesthesia is used to block both the nerves and nerve endings. It can be directed to a specific nerve by injection or applied to the skin as a gel or via an impregnated cloth. The duration of effect varies with the type of anesthetic and may last for many hours with long-acting local anesthetics.

Neuroablation. Neuroablation is the destruction of a nerve that is identified as the cause of severe, intractable pain, such as neuralgia resulting from injury to the intercostal nerves during chest or upper abdominal surgery. Toxic agents such as alcohol or phenol can be injected into targeted nerves; in other cases, *cryoanalgesia* (freezing) or *radiofrequency ablation* (heating by radiofrequency energy) can destroy the nerve tissues.

Intradiscal Electrotherapy. As an alternative to surgery, intradiscal electrotherapy (IDET) is a recently introduced technique that targets pain caused by degenerative changes in spinal disks. A needle is inserted into the affected disk, allowing a small heated cannula to be introduced. The heat produced not only blocks pain signals from small nerves in the disk wall, but also may seal cracks in the disk. But just because new pain-management techniques are available, it does not mean that they are better than older methods. Until a technique has been rigorously studied for many years in thousands of patients, it is unlikely to be validated by evidence-based medicine. It is best to stay with the tried-and-true in most cases. Your pain-management specialist can recommend the therapy most likely to be effective.

Intradiscal Bicuplasty. Another nonsurgical technique developed from the early experience with minimally invasive spinal procedures is intradiscal bicuplasty. This technique, which uses two needles and has all the safeguards to prevent any nerve damage, has been validated and may offer the best long-term results of all these recent nonsurgical spinal therapies for chronic disk pain.

Neuromodulation

When pain no longer responds to medications delivered by any route or to any other measures, neuromodulation techniques are considered. These techniques are primarily reserved for neuropathic pain and include spinal cord stimulation, peripheral nerve stimulation, and deep brain stimulation. Typically, patients go through a psychological assessment and then a trial period stimulation to make sure that this option is right for them. Sixteen-year-old Bobbie was one such patient.

Bobbie

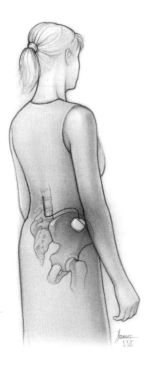

Because of congenital abnormalities in both feet, Bobbie had undergone many surgeries to correct the deformities. A major nerve in one foot had been damaged during one of the operations and she developed complex regional pain syndrome/reflex sympathetic dystrophy. Bobbie's symptoms were localized in her foot and ankle, which were very, very sensitive to the touch. Medications had not helped at all, so eventually Bobbie sought help from Cleveland Clinic pain specialists. A spinal cord stimulator was used on a trial basis, and it worked so well in reducing Bobbie's level of pain that it was later implanted. Today, Bobbie attends college and maintains nearly normal activities, which had been impossible before.

The pulse generator (shown) can be implanted in a pocket beneath the hip bone (iliac crest), with the electrode (shown) entering the spine in the lower back.

Spinal cord stimulation involves implanting a small, programmable generator into a pocket created under the skin. This pain pacemaker sends low-level electricity through leads placed near affected nerve fibers in the space above the spinal cord. Sending electrical impulses directly to the pain source creates a buzzing or tingling sensation that interferes with the transmission of pain signals. The result is that painful neuropathies become much more manageable and the affected extremity can respond to physical and occupational therapy.

Complementary and Alternative Medicine

Today, 22 million Americans use complementary and alternative therapies to treat pain and other symptoms. It's a huge industry. The use of alternative therapies has grown from $11 billion in 1991 to $14 billion in 2009.

About 100 therapies are categorized as *mind-body interventions*. Some of these holistic methods of healing pain date from thousands of years ago, and some are recent innovations. They embrace manual healing or massage, herbal medicine, lifestyle diets (macrobiotics), energy healing, magnetic therapy, homeopathy, and folk remedies. Some methods, such as acupuncture and transcutaneous electrical nerve stimulation, are well-established remedies for controlling specific types of pain.

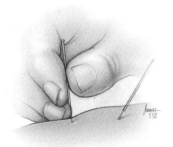

Acupuncture. Acupuncture is an ancient Chinese practice that involves inserting fine needles into selected points on the skin that

Acupuncture

correspond to specific pain states. Today, it is used to relieve the pain of peripheral neuropathy, cancer, or arthritis.

Transcutaneous Electrical Nerve Stimulation. Transcutaneous electrical nerve stimulation (TENS) is a means of delivering electrical energy to nerve fibers in the spine. A battery-powered device, worn externally, sends electrical impulses through electrodes placed over painful sites. People have used TENS to manage migraine, arthritis, shingles, and sciatica.

Biofeedback. Biofeedback helps us become aware of and control the body's response to pain. Using equipment that senses nervous system arousal (such as changes in skin temperature and electrical activity in muscles), participants learn to relax muscles voluntarily to prevent migraines, for instance.

Meditation and Guided Imagery. Relaxation techniques such as meditation or guided imagery effectively ease headache pain without medication.

• • • *Fast Fact* • • •

The National Center for Complementary and Alternative Medicine, a division of the National Institutes of Health, researches the safety and efficacy of the increasingly popular alternative therapies. (Visit *http://nccam.nih.gov* for more information.)

• • •

Hypnosis. Hypnosis, when employed by skilled practitioners, can serve as a useful adjunct to conventional treatment in relieving pain and disability.

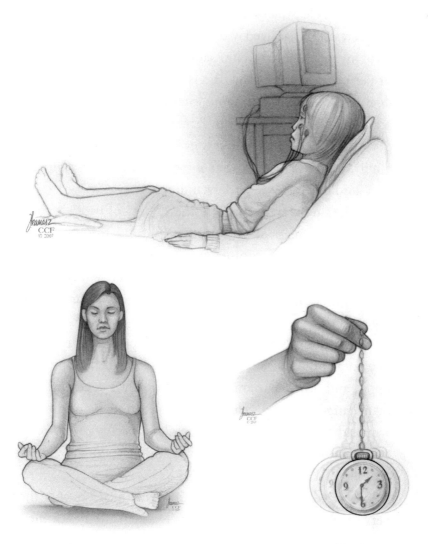

Complementary and alternative therapies to treat pain include biofeedback (top), relaxation techniques such as meditation (lower left), and hypnosis (lower right).

The Power of Positive Thinking (and Prayer)

Last but not least, let's not ignore the power of positive thinking. Teresa, 35, has lived with pain since her childhood diagnosis of juvenile arthritis. Now saddled with the added diagnosis of peripheral neuropathy, she is in pain day and night. No doctor could help her; some even accused her of trying to scam them for pain pills. Yet Teresa remains optimistic.

When asked why, she rattles off a long list: friends and family, a support group she's joined, God, exercise, medication, and a new, more understanding doctor.

There's no way to measure the impact of positive thinking on a person's pain or condition. But one thing is certain: Doing nothing but complaining only increases pain symptoms and associated disabilities. The more active we are in our bodies and our minds, the more likely we are to set forth on the road to recovery.

Then there is that mysterious and potent intervention known as prayer. Jack was 47 years old when he injured his upper and lower extremities in a terrible car accident. After many surgeries, he developed severe, burning pain in his left arm and to a lesser extent in both legs. Jack was referred to a pain clinic and diagnosed with complex regional pain syndrome (CRPS).

He tried antiseizure drugs and pain medications, then nerve and spinal cord stimulation. Disenchanted with medical approaches, he consulted a faith healer, figuring it couldn't hurt. After four months of visits, Jack no longer had any symptoms in his arm or legs. His implanted stimulators were removed, and one year later he remained free of CRPS.

Hope is a small word packed with powerful meaning. When you hope, you have something upon which to construct a life. In learning to live productively in the face of chronic pain, people discover renewed hope for themselves.

A Sample Pain Program

This daily schedule, adapted from one created by the University of Washington Pain Center, where Doctors Bonica and Fordyce worked, illustrates the structure of a typical week in a pain program.

Monday–Friday morning

8:00–8:25 A.M.	Movement, stretch, and body mechanics
8:35–10:35 A.M.	Physical and occupational therapy (individual and group sessions)
10:45–11:15 A.M.	Skill-building groups
11:15–11:45 A.M.	Relaxation and muscle reeducation sessions

Monday–Friday afternoon

12:00–12:30 P.M.	Lunch
12:15–12:55 P.M.	Treatment-team rounds
12:30–12:55 P.M.	Muscle reeducation (individual sessions)
1:00–1:50 P.M.	MD didactic lecture group (physician instruction)

2:00–2:55 P.M.	Physical and occupational therapy (individual and group sessions)
3:00–3:15 P.M.	Psychology didactic group (psychologist instruction)
4:00–4:55 P.M.	Physical therapy (individual sessions)

Saturday morning

8:30–9:30 A.M.	Group physical therapy
9:30–10:30 A.M.	Group occupational therapy
10:30–11:00 A.M.	Group stretch class

Chapter 7

When a Child Is in Pain

I n October 2005, the International Association for the Study of Pain (IASP) declared a Global Year Against Pain in Children to call attention to worldwide undertreatment of acute and chronic pain in the young. While data on chronic pain in children is sparse, we know that chronic pain affects a child's family relationships, school attendance, participation in extracurricular activities, friendships, and ability to fulfill responsibilities at home. Children in chronic pain easily fall prey to feelings of sadness, anxiety, isolation, frustration, and anger. This takes a heavy toll on parents, who struggle to cope with their child's predicament, and on the child's siblings.

Because a child's pain so completely alters family dynamics and will have a profound impact on the child's future life, the pediatric psychologist plays an indispensable role on the pain-care team. A 2008 report by the International Association for the Study of Pain stated that a substantial body of research showed that cognitive and behavioral techniques used by psychologists can effectively reduce pain and distress in children having invasive procedures. These techniques become even more valuable when applied to treatments for chronic pain.

Sarah

While being chased by a girl at school, 12-year-old Sarah smacked her forefinger on a desk. It immediately began to swell; she'd whacked it really hard. The initial injury was treated as a ligament strain and a bruise. But over the next three months, the swelling progressed to involve Sarah's entire hand, wrist, and forearm. Her skin was discolored, bluish, and cold to the touch. She was diagnosed with complex regional pain syndrome/regional sympathetic dystrophy. After six months of physical and occupational therapy, along with antiseizure and pain medications, feeling in Sarah's arm and hand had not improved. Her hand was especially sensitive to pain.

It was determined that the probable source of Sarah's pain was a dysfunction of her sympathetic nervous system. This system regulates our fight-or-flight response, triggering changes in blood-vessel size and heart rate, among other things. Sarah's parents agreed to a sympathetic nerve block.

Under X-ray guidance, an anesthetic was injected near a group of nerves known as the stellate ganglion, which transmits pain signals to the arm and hand. As soon as her sympathetic nervous system activity was interrupted, Sarah sat up in bed and smiled. Her symptoms had

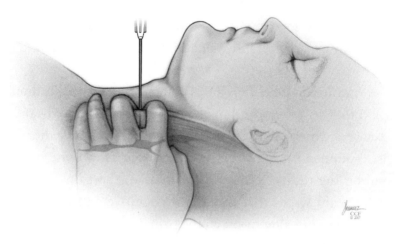

Figure shows a needle positioned to inject a local anesthetic near the sympathetic nerves (stellate ganglion).

virtually disappeared. That sympathetic block gave Sarah a period of freedom from pain that allowed her to resume occupational therapy. She regained her hand function and developed a good grip.

To help Sarah achieve long-term pain relief, her rehabilitation plan called for psychological intervention. She attended cognitive and behavioral therapy sessions with a pediatric clinical psychologist trained to help children manage their pain symptoms. Within four months, her symptoms had completely disappeared.

Knowledge Is Power

Many psychological pitfalls serve as unwanted baggage on a child's journey through chronic pain. Though many parents are reluctant to seek the help of mental-health professionals for fear of stigmatizing their children, an understanding of the pain experience and its natural effects on children and teens can be empowering.

A common stereotype holds that children complain about pain to gain attention, but the truth is that children rarely exaggerate their pain. When behavioral and cognitive therapy is recommended for children or adolescents, no one is disputing the reality of their pain. Instead, the pain-management team hopes that the use of cognitive and behavioral techniques can alter or lessen the pain experience. The idea is to help children function at their best by eliminating any pain magnified by stress, anxiety, and depression.

As one pediatric psychologist explains, "A tension headache is a real headache, and it may have a physiological, or organic, cause. But it's my job to determine whether other factors—psychological, environmental, sociological, stress-related—are 'cranking up the volume' of that pain."

For example, a teen with recurrent tension headaches may be trying to keep up with academically challenging courses without missing choir rehearsals or skipping volleyball practice—all the while holding down a part-time job. Soon, the teen's cup is overflowing with activities.

No matter how fulfilling these activities may be, that teen is in a pressure-cooker. Could the teen's overburdened lifestyle be a factor in recurrent tension headaches? Certainly.

Learning Pain Behaviors

Children can learn pain behaviors just as adults do. When any of us experiences pain for a long period, we may adopt the learned pain response outlined by Dr. Fordyce. For example, when we develop a painful sinus infection, we continue to anticipate waking up in pain even after the antibiotics have taken hold.

In just this way, children learn to anticipate pain that has persisted for a long time. Some children worry that they will never get better, and they cannot envision a pain-free future.

A child's anxiety is unsurprising when everyone around him shows constant concern. Repeatedly asking children how they feel, for example, can frighten them by making them focus on their pain.

In addition, parents can inadvertently perpetuate a child's symptoms if the child grows accustomed to receiving special treatment. When pain episodes cause children to stay home from school and avoid chores, parents may try to cheer them by allowing them to watch television, surf the Web, or play video games. Children can grow reluctant to give up these privileges, reinforcing pain behaviors.

Evaluation of the Child in Pain

A low-key approach to determining how much pain a child feels is always best, but assessing pain in children can be difficult, particularly in younger children. Children do not display the same physical signs of pain as adults, such as elevated blood pressure or heart rate. So diagnosing a child's pain becomes more a matter of reading signs than anything else.

These are common indicators that a child is experiencing pain:

- **Infants.** An infant in pain will cry and cannot be soothed by feeding, changing, or being held.

- **Toddlers.** Often a toddler's pain masquerades as fussiness or irritability. A Cleveland Clinic pediatric psychologist notes, "Their vocabulary is limited, and this inability to verbalize can frustrate them. While lab findings are being assessed, we can ask toddlers in a concrete way if something is feeling 'yucky' or 'achy'—without planting the idea in their minds."

- **Preschoolers.** Because of their naturally happy and curious natures, preschoolers in pain are particularly hard to read. In fact, their pain experience may be less than that of an older child who has the same organic cause of pain.

- **School-age children.** An older child's perception of pain is more in line with an adult's. Children of school age are much more able to talk about their pain.

Different Ages, Different Pain

Age and temperament affect the type of pain a child experiences and its intensity. Pain tends to be less overwhelming for an easygoing child, while a child who is clingy or a worrier may experience more pain. For example:

- Recurrent stomachaches are typically seen in children with true anxiety disorders or situational anxiety.

- Vague somatic complaints, along the lines of "something just doesn't feel right," are typical of middle-school-age children.

- Recurrent headaches, both tension and migraine, are the most common pain problem in older adolescents. They tend to develop in high-achievers who take academics seriously, set high standards for themselves and others, and don't cope well with situations or individuals who don't meet those expectations.

Measuring a Child's Pain

Measuring how much pain a patient is feeling is critical to determining how well a pain-management technique is working. Because children and adolescents vary in their ability to express their pain, pain specialists use different measures to assess their pain.

In younger children, the FACES pain scale is used to rate pain levels. The simply drawn faces on the chart, ranging in expression from happy to sad, correspond to different levels of pain.

Older children are able to report their level of pain. However, psychological factors can intervene. For example, an adolescent with sickle-cell anemia may develop anticipatory anxiety due to a past pain crisis, as the episodes are called, and worry that the oncoming pain will be just as severe. The anxiety may make the teen rate his or her current pain as 10 on the pain scale, when in reality it is more likely an 8. It's hard to tease apart the difference in these cases.

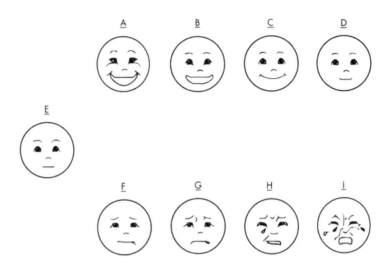

The FACES pain scale is used to rate pain levels in younger children.

Measurement of pain levels is used throughout treatment and rehabilitation by the pain-management team. For psychologists, the measurements track the efficacy of tools such as positive self-talk, deep breathing, progressive muscle relaxation, and guided imagery.

Tools for Pediatric Pain Treatment

In contrast to adults, children are more compliant and respond better to behavioral measures and physical modalities. Children's pain will often respond to weak analgesics, anti-inflammatories, anticonvulsants, and antidepressants. Integrated programs of rehabilitation that include biofeedback, physical therapy, swimming, music therapy, and concurrent schooling are most effective for treating children's pain.

The Power of Self-Talk. "A big part of my work is help-ing patients and families to think differently about pain, to reward and reinforce healthy behaviors, to remain neutral about negative pain behaviors, and to encourage positive self-talk," says a Cleveland Clinic pediatric psychologist.

Positive self-talk is a powerful tool. Children in pain can develop a habit of talking to themselves positively about their situation: "Yes, I know I have this problem. But I'm not going to let it stop me from getting out of bed and going to school today. If I go to school today, my friends will be happy to see me and I won't get behind in my schoolwork."

Another self-talk scenario might be: "I know nothing scary is going on inside me. Even though I have this big disease, it is manageable over time. I trust my doctors and I'm going to help myself get through this."

The Art of Distraction. Drawing a child's attention away from his or her pain by focusing the child's attention on other activities is a worthwhile endeavor. Children and adolescents who have been inactive for a period of time can become reen-gaged through *activity cycling.* This involves performing an activity for ten minutes, then taking a five-minute break, then doing a different activity. The idea is to develop a cycle of activity instead of lying on the couch.

Taking a Deep Breath. Teaching children about deep breath-ing, or breathing from the diaphragm, is an easy way to help children learn to relax themselves. Pediatric psychologists may work with children before they start chemotherapy to help them relax enough to control any nausea. "As soon as the pain begins creeping up, I tell kids it's like filling up a giant balloon

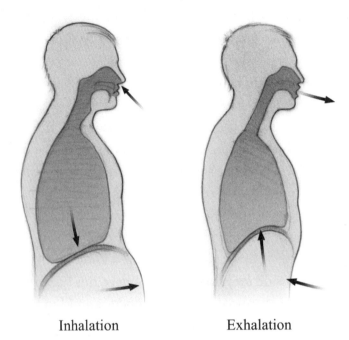

Inhalation   Exhalation

in your belly. You fill it up, then blow a giant bubble through a bubble wand and let it out," says one psychologist.

The science behind this technique is that diaphragmatic breathing brings a healthy influx of oxygen into your body. When oxygen flows through the body, it has a calming affect.

Progressive Relaxation. Remember when you were a kid and you tackled the monkey bars fearlessly? Your large muscle groups would work hard to help you negotiate the span, bar by bar, until you grasped the top rung. Then you'd collapse to the ground, your muscles like jelly.

Progressive muscle relaxation works in a similar way. The child isolates the major muscle groups one at a time, beginning with the toes, tensing each set of muscles for

Basic Diaphragmatic Breathing:
Sample Script for a Child with Headache

(Developed to Help a Child Relax at the ONSET of a Headache)

One of the first things we are going to work on is breathing. We know that you know how to breathe. But the way you breathe—actually, the way we all breathe day to day—is not the best type of breathing to help get rid of your headaches.

Have you ever seen how young babies or animals breathe? If you watch them closely, you'll see that they don't seem to breathe with their chest or shoulders, but rather, with their stomach area. They don't suck in their abdomens but actually expand their bellies as they breathe in, using the muscle at the bottom of their lungs, the diaphragm. Their shoulders and other large muscles stay relaxed. (See diagram on opposite page.) That's what you are going to do. It sounds easy, but for most people it takes practice. It tends to feel like you are doing something wrong at first, because it's so different from what you are used to.

Let me show you. I start by relaxing my shoulders and chest area. I breathe in through my nose, trying to fill up the bottom of my lungs first, almost as if I'm pouring water into a big balloon, filling up the bottom first. As my lungs fill from the bottom up, my stomach area expands, and my lungs gradually fill up to the top of my chest. Then I let the air out through my mouth with a soft "whoooo" sound. Let's try it.

Start by sitting comfortably, legs not crossed and arms on the arms of the chair. Relax your shoulders and neck. Take a deep breath in through your nose, filling up from the bottom of your lungs. Good ... Fill them all the way up, keeping your shoulders relaxed. Good! Now slowly let the air out, like collapsing a balloon. Good! Let's try another.

How do you feel? Some people feel a bit dizzy at first, with such a rush of oxygen to their systems. That will go

(continued)

away in a few seconds. Can you feel the relaxed feeling in your shoulders and chest? Good.

Jensen, V. K. and Yaldoo, D. T. (2000), "Basic Diaphragmatic Breathing Sample Script," in "Assessment and Treatment of Chronic Headaches in Adolescents." *Innovations in Clinical Practice: A Source Book* (V. 18), Sarasota, FL: Professional Resource Exchange, Inc. Copyright © 2000 by Professional Resource Exchange, Inc. Reprinted by permission.

ten seconds and then relaxing them for ten, slowly moving up the body all the way to the scalp.

Guided Imagery. Children are especially responsive to guided imagery—techniques that help us imagine ourselves in a happy or peaceful place. They need to focus on something that gives them a nice, relaxed feeling. A 9-year-old girl might imagine swimming with dolphins. A 14-year-old boy might imagine darting through defenders on the football field, pivoting left and right to the end zone. The goal is for children to picture themselves in a happy setting when they close their eyes, breathe deeply, and talk through what they are imagining. Adults may need recorded sounds of the ocean or rain during guided imagery sessions, but children generally need nothing more than their imaginations. Most children are responsive to positive self-talk, deep breathing, progressive muscle relaxation, and guided imagery. Those who may be reluctant at the outset generally become willing to try the techniques. Some may not be able to translate that willingness into action. Still others are reluctant even to set foot in the psychologist's office, which is why in a multidisciplinary setting most children will be active participants.

Pain Diaries and Patterns

For children who are completely open to interacting with a psychologist, a pain diary can be enormously useful.

Keeping a pain diary allows patterns to emerge that wouldn't necessarily be identified during an individual session. In logging their pain, children note:

- The pain sensation
- Its intensity
- Its location
- Its timing
- The circumstances

For example, when five of a child's last seven headaches occurred right after the child finished doing math homework, it suggests that something related to that activity needs to be addressed.

Best Practices for Parents

Parents should fully support their child's participation in cognitive and behavioral therapy, and participate themselves when asked.

When pain develops, they can gently encourage their child to employ positive self-talk, relaxation techniques, and other techniques to alleviate symptoms. If children can't go to school, parents should have them rest quietly in bed as they would with any illness, rather than allow them unrestricted access to the computer and television.

It's healthiest for children to attend school, take part in extracurricular activities, and enjoy their friendships as much as possible. It's also important to expect children to keep up with chores. This sends a positive signal that parents see their child as strong enough to manage the pain.

When a child withdraws from friends during severe pain episodes, parents can step in and suggest activities that they can pursue together that will engage the child and divert attention from the pain.

Pediatric Palliative Medicine

Some children experience pain while in the throes of a terminal illness such as cancer. Nothing is as heartbreaking as watching a child die. To meet the needs of their pediatric patients, a good pain-management team has an anesthesiologist working with the child's family physician, oncologist, or other specialists, along with therapists, nurses, and social workers. A key member of this team is the pediatric palliative-medicine specialist.

Anesthesiologists can keep a child comfortable through a variety of local and regional pain-management techniques. A psychologist trained in pediatric palliative medicine uses other tools to help a child through the end of life. Ideally, the psychologist is brought in early enough to develop a relationship with the dying child and his or her family.

Pediatric psychologists work with many young cancer patients, serving as medical interpreters who help child and family understand what is happening and help families cope with death and bereavement issues.

Young Heroes

Despite the devastating circumstances associated with terminally ill young children, examples of heroic behavior by those children abound. One of the biggest rewards for doctors who help children through terminal illness is witnessing their strength and resiliency.

Despite our best efforts to make children comfortable, pain cannot always be fully controlled. "Yet children can be full of life and energy despite their pain," says one doctor. "They teach us so many lessons about how to live."

Chapter 8

Pain in the Elderly and End-of-Life Care

*"Effective pain and symptom management is an ethical obligation for all health-care providers and organizations…
We have the knowledge and ability to deliver skillful and effective control of pain and suffering at the end of life."*
—American Academy of Pain Medicine
Position Statement (1989)

Individuals who are 85 and older are the fastest growing segment of the U.S. population. As the average American lifespan lengthens, the challenge posed by chronic pain poses an ever greater challenge to the pain-management specialists tasked with treating the condition. It is believed that about four-fifths of the elderly in the United States live with at least one painful chronic condition. They may suffer the musculoskeletal pain of arthritis or backache, the neuropathic pain of diabetes or shingles, or the circulatory pain of atherosclerosis or thrombophlebitis. And let's not forget cancer and the other diseases to which the elderly so easily fall prey.

Not having the multitude of distractions that can influence the severity of pain in younger individuals, it is necessary to appreciate its impact on the elderly by treating chronic pain effectively.

Difficult Circumstances

The guarding behaviors that Dr. Fordyce described are of particular concern with elderly patients. When the elderly guard painful joints and muscles, it not only aggravates pain resulting from disuse, as it does in younger patients, but it also contributes to a decline in their functional independence and overall mobility.

Any loss of function or mobility drastically impairs the quality of life for independent-minded elderly individuals as disability renders them homebound and socially isolated. To become more dependent on others for basic needs distresses—and depresses—many senior citizens.

To complicate matters, many elderly people must take several medications, each of which can interact with the others as well as with over-the-counter medicines, producing mental confusion. This unfortunately sets the stage for an elderly patient, without realizing the problem, to take incorrect amounts of prescribed medicines. Further complicating matters is that approximately 47 percent of people over age 85 meet the criteria for Alzheimer's disease. The end result? A dangerous mix of frail elderly individuals, often with impaired ability to comprehend and communicate, attempting to care for themselves and deal with painful infirmities.

Home Care and Pain Management

Most aging people live in their homes rather than in skilled nursing facilities, and most are on fixed incomes. When it comes to managing a senior patient's pain, home care is an affordable alternative. In 2009, home health care averaged $30 per hour, while hospital care averaged a cost of $125 per hour.

Families considering home care for aging relatives with chronic pain must make careful choices. We adapted the following guidelines from John S. Spratt's *Home Health Care: Principles and Practices,* and added a few of our own:

- The patient must want health-care services at home, the home environment must be conducive to home care, and the patient must be able to pay for it. Obviously, the patient's medical state should be sufficiently stable to warrant home care.

- The patient must understand that total pain relief may be unrealistic—and that the goal is control, rather than elimination, of pain.

- A pain-management specialist should oversee the patient's care and be available to evaluate the patient's condition frequently.

- The patient or caregiver must fully understand medication doses and side effects, know how to manage adverse reactions, and be able to procure and dispose of prescriptions properly.

- The caregiver must be able troubleshoot problems with home-care devices, maintain equipment, manage alarms, and respect device limitations.

- Pain relief must be accompanied by an acceptable level of function. For example, the dose of medication from an infusion pump should not interfere with a patient's ability to communicate or, if he or she is able, to get around.

As described throughout this book, the most effective, safe, and compassionate care for people in pain requires a coalition of individuals and agencies. Moreover, a smooth operation depends upon good communication among the patient, physician, home-care providers, pharmacy, hospital, and health insurers.

Finding Certified Care Providers

Home health agencies and hospices must be certified by Medicare, and many city, county, and state departments for the aging offer Medicare-certified home health care.

To meet Joint Commission on Accreditation of Healthcare Organizations (JCAHO) accreditation for home health care, an agency must offer:

- Home-care equipment services
- Nursing; physical, speech, and occupational therapy; nutrition services; and social-work support
- Custodial care services
- Pharmaceutical and respiratory care

U.S. home care agencies employ more than 500,000 caregivers. Most caregivers are home care aides, and some are registered nurses or licensed practical nurses (LPNs). Physical and occupational therapists, social workers, and speech pathologists also play a key role on any home care team.

Many outreach programs that support home care are based at regional hospitals or local physician group practices. This is as it should be, considering most homebound elderly do not live near skilled nursing facilities or large medical centers. Today, home health care is widely available even in rural areas.

Hospital Services at Home

Pharmacological pain control can be provided in the home. In addition, the special pain-management techniques deployed in hospitals can be provided at home by visiting nurses following strict protocols. Portable pumps can deliver analgesics under the skin, into the epidural space surrounding the spinal cord, or into the intrathecal space surrounding the brain and spinal cord.

How and where pain medication is administered depends upon the character and intensity of the elderly patient's pain, as well as the patient's physical status and immune-system integrity. The nurse's ability to provide patient education and the social structure within the home are other factors to be weighed. Finally, the visiting nurse's experience with a particular technique and the frequency of home visits must be evaluated.

With the increasing sophistication of infusion pumps, patients can enjoy far greater freedom than was the case with older pumps. In addition, the pumps save time and money because they require patients to make fewer visits to the hospital or doctor's office. While good communication between patient and physician remains critical, newer pumps can store their usage histories digitally, so they can be transmitted via telemetry directly to the physician's office over the phone.

Palliative Medicine

Chronic pain should be managed so it doesn't interfere with activities of daily living or with the quality of the patient's life. But the need to manage pain is just as urgent, if not more so, for the dying. In other words, at the end of life.

The end of life is defined as approximately the six-month period preceding an anticipated death. Providing pain management and comfort care in the hospital at the end of life is called *palliative medicine,* and it is a large part of what we do.

Most Americans die in an institutional setting, such as a hospital or long-term care facility. But growing evidence suggests that home care services offer a viable option for patients who wish to spend their last days in their homes. There is no reason why patients who have done well with an external infusion system in the hospital cannot go home. Ambulatory infusion pumps serve a number of purposes besides pain management: they can deliver antibiotics, hydration therapy, and nutrition at the same time.

Home-care agencies can support dying patients who rely on external systems or implanted pumps for pain control, refilling pump reservoirs with medications as needed. This gives dying patients substantial freedom from pain and affords them the opportunity for close contact with loved ones in familiar surroundings.

Jane, Revisited

In chapter 3 we met Jane, who had developed a bleeding ulcer from overuse of ibuprofen and was hospitalized for gastric surgery. Initially, her recovery went well, but then she began to deteriorate and contracted pneumonia. Jane's breathing became labored, and tests revealed a pulmonary embolism, a dangerous clot blocking blood flow to her lungs.

In response to Jane's breathing problems, her doctors put her on a ventilator. She managed to come off the ventilator a few days later and breathe on her own. But after she was transferred to a step-down unit, Jane's breathing again grew labored. Tests revealed another pulmonary embolism. Ominously, this time she showed signs of congestive heart failure as well.

Jane had a living will, which clearly documented that she did not want to be kept alive by artificial means. Faced with the gravity of her condition, Jane's family and her doctors decided to bring in hospice.

Hospice workers are skilled in offering emotional support for the dying person as well as the family. Jane's large family gathered around her, making sure she was comfortable at all times. The hospice nurse sat with the family and explained the types of medications Jane was receiving and how they worked to keep her comfortable.

The nurse also took time to compassionately explain what was happening physically to Jane's body as her systems began to shut down, one by one. This was comfort care not just for Jane, but for her whole family.

Needless Suffering

What people nearing death fear more than dying itself is needless suffering. In 2000, the *Journal of the American Medical Association* reported on a survey of seriously ill patients, recently bereaved families, physicians, and other care providers. Researchers hoped to identify key factors influencing quality end-of-life care. Despite individual differences and roles, most respondents agreed that management of pain and symptoms was one of several key factors influencing good care at the end of life.

Unfortunately, pain remains vastly undertreated in America, even at the end of life. A still timely 2001 *Journal of the American Medical Association* survey found that 14 percent of all nursing home residents reported persistent pain. When reassessed 60 to 180 days later, 40 percent of the same group had developed severe pain.

Consider these additional statistics:

- In 1997, a time when many landmark pain studies were conducted, researchers reported in the *Annals of Internal Medicine* that 40 percent of people who die in the United States die in pain. That same year, the National Academy of Sciences Institute of Medicine reported that 40 to 80 percent of terminally ill patients received inadequate treatment for pain.
- The National Cancer Policy Board, a committee of the Institute of Medicine and the National Research Council, has stated that half the 550,000 Americans who die from cancer each year needlessly suffer from pain, nausea, depression, fatigue, and other discomfort.

In the face of such institutional apathy, the American Psychological Association asserted that people in pain have the right to expect pain relief and that pain relief should be a priority. In June 1997, the U.S. Supreme Court formally ruled that the medical profession has a responsibility to relieve patients' pain and suffering. This ruling has been adopted and written into the legislature of most states.

Pain Care Bill of Rights

The American Pain Foundation sums up the rights of individuals who are in pain in this way:

As a person with pain, you have:

- The right to have your report of pain taken seriously and to be treated with dignity and respect by doctors, nurses, pharmacists, and other health-care professionals
- The right to have your pain thoroughly assessed and promptly treated
- The right to be informed by your doctor about what may be causing your pain, possible treatments, and the benefits, risks, and costs of each
- The right to participate actively in decisions about how to manage your pain
- The right to have your pain reassessed regularly and your treatment adjusted if your pain has not been eased
- The right to be referred to a pain specialist if your pain persists
- The right to receive clear and prompt answers to your questions, to take time to make decisions, and to refuse a particular type of treatment if you choose

The mission statement of the American Pain Foundation is as follows:

The American Pain Foundation is an independent nonprofit 501(c)(3) organization serving people with pain through information, advocacy, and support. Our mission is to improve the quality of life of people with pain by raising public awareness, providing practical information, promoting research, and advocating to remove barriers and increase access to effective pain management.

Chapter 9

Raising Awareness, Building Legislation

Twenty-nine years ago, Penny Cowan spent seven weeks in Cleveland Clinic's Chronic Pain Rehabilitation Program (see chapter 6). Ever since, she has continued to walk through the doors that began to open for her. Penny eventually wrote a book about her experiences, *Patient or Person: Living with Chronic Pain.*

When her rehabilitation ended, she was concerned. "I knew I could handle the pain in the controlled environment of the pain clinic. During the drive home I wasn't so sure the routine could work at home."

But Penny continued to rely on the biofeedback training and other therapies she had received at the clinic. "I'm able to listen and respond to what my body is telling me. My pain is a part of me, but it isn't my identity," she says.

Penny notes that the determining question is always, "Do we have more reason to stay sick or to get better? I had a lot to gain by getting better."

Her pain has not gone, but it no longer dominates her life. "I'm in every sense of the word a person. I don't think of myself as a patient or as disabled. I don't focus on my physical well-being. I don't focus on it, so I don't suffer. The pain is there, but it's not controlling me," she says.

If Penny learned anything in the pain clinic, it was that she was not alone. So she started a support group at her church to share what she had learned with others. "I didn't want the support group to be about who was feeling worse or who had died. I knew there were others like me who suffered but didn't necessarily show it, because pain is invisible."

This led to Penny giving talks and being interviewed for newspaper stories. Eventually, seven other support groups arose in the Pittsburgh area. Today, Penny's little support group has grown into the American Chronic Pain Association.

With headquarters in Rocklin, California, the foundation has spawned hundreds of support groups across the United States, Canada, and Great Britain. The organization focuses on providing peer support, coping skills, and resources. Penny is executive director.

Now a grandmother of two, she still gets up every morning and does the stretches she learned at the Cleveland Clinic so long ago. She puts in a full day, developing education programs and talking to individuals who are in pain.

"I want to reach out to the people sitting there, waiting and hoping as I did. I want them to know that first, they are not alone, and second, there is hope and there are ways to gain control," she says. "We are survivors. Not giving up is part of the human spirit."

Tackling Chronic Pain at the National Level

Public policies on treatment, reimbursement, and research for chronic pain have not made it any easier for people in pain to find relief, according to Will Rowe, executive director of the American Pain Foundation.

There is no national consensus on what constitutes appropriate care for chronic pain. Yet we ignore the issue of chronic pain at our financial peril. The social costs reach into the tens of billions of dollars annually, most often from lost worker productivity. Pain causes more disability in America than cancer and heart disease combined. Accounting for 20 percent of medical visits per year, pain is the second most common reason given for seeing a doctor; 86 million Americans have visited a doctor at least once for pain lasting one month or longer. In fact, the Obama administration is currently planning to concentrate on the clinical outcomes of most clinical treatments with a view to reducing the economic and health impact of those treatments having poor or questionable results.

Our society is poorly equipped to help those suffering with chronic pain, according to the American Chronic Pain Association. They document some sobering statistics:

- Of pain patients surveyed, three in ten have been unable to get a prescription filled because of cost or lack of insurance.

- Nearly three in ten believe that it will become more difficult to get the medication they will need in the future.

- Too few resources exist for those who don't have medical insurance through their employer; private insurance is expensive and often has onerous restrictions or no coverage, particularly because of preexisting conditions.

- Doctors are reluctant to prescribe adequate pain medication even to patients they've known for years because of concern over increasing tolerance, addiction, respiratory depression, illicit use, and regulatory action.

A Look at Workplace Injuries

To examine the shortcomings of our public policies on chronic-pain care, consider how workplace injuries are handled. The workplace is the site of many injuries that trigger intractable pain. About 40 percent of my own caseload is made up of work-related injuries, a common statistic among pain specialists. We are often called upon to defend those who are denied treatment for one reason or another. The amount of "office time" (representing telephone communication with third party payers including the Bureau of Workers' Compensation), dictation, and/or transcription in a 55-hour workweek is at least 15 percent.

The Bureau of Workers' Compensation (BWC) does not yet recognize that the majority of injured people want to get well and return to work as quickly as possible. Adding to the complexity of the situation are those who argue that injured parties who make claims are seeking a large settlement against big business or the BWC—an adversarial view that sees everyone as thirsting for the highest payout. In reality, only a relatively small percentage of patients want to bleed the system.

Further complicating matters are the lawyers who doggedly pursue cases through the courts, spending money on this broken system instead of on an injured patient's care and recovery. As injured workers wait through the appeals process to learn whether their claims will be paid, months can pass.

What's the Danger of Delaying Treatment?

Delaying treatment can turn a relatively minor injury into a major health problem. A rapid response to back injury in the workplace, for example, can prevent the development of chronic pain in many cases. While injured workers wait in limbo for the outcome of a workers' compensation decision or appeal, their very livelihoods can be jeopardized.

Supervised physical therapy is a crucial element of rehabilitation and can be the determining factor in a patient's return to work or eligibility for vocational training. About 70 to 80 percent of patients need three to six months of therapy, which must be supervised to prevent reinjury from improperly executed movements.

But, frustratingly, most health plans do not cover rehabilitation for the entire length of time required, and Medicare or Medicaid will not provide coverage until a patient is 65 years old or destitute. Many injured workers end up paying out of pocket and are financially drained. Others simply never complete the rehabilitative therapy they need for optimal functioning in life.

If Most Patients Want to Return to Work, Why Does It Seem as Though People on Disability Rarely Do?

Most physicians will tell you that among the first few questions a patient asks following a workplace injury is, "When can I go back to work?" The truth is, when problems arise, they happen precisely *because* of the delays that the Bureau of Workers' Compensation system cultivates. Six months is the magic period. Once a patient has been on disability for six months, his or her chances of going back to work decline dramatically. That may be why people who are self-employed seem to do better in rehabilitation than those who are employees. Because self-employed people are the masters of their own destinies and have no choice, they may work harder at their recovery and be less likely to wait for their cases to move through the system.

Moreover, sometimes Social Security Income can foster the sick role mentioned earlier. If you cannot reclaim the job or economic position you held before you were injured, you may begin—without even realizing it—to look for ways to extend the payouts.

A large part of how you deal with pain depends upon your personality. Pain looms as a much larger factor for a dependent personality than for a driven Type A personality. Take a trucker who earns $75,000 to $100,000 a year driving a big rig, but then finds himself living on $20,000 a year in disability income. A more dependent personality may look at that lifestyle and prefer remaining sick to working. But a Type A personality may be driven to work hard during rehabilitation to reclaim the life he once led.

Fixing the System

The United States turns a cold shoulder to injured workers, compared with other countries that take a more compassionate approach. Australia, for example, has no-fault insurance that kicks in to cover rehabilitation and income for injured workers.

People who sustain industrial injuries in the United Kingdom, Germany, and Switzerland experience a much less adversarial environment than do workers who are similarly injured in America.

As a first step toward improving the system in the United States, beginning the arbitration process at the time of injury might serve a role similar to that of triage in the emergency setting. Assembling the appropriate experts at the outset—orthopedists, internists, and/or anesthesiologists—would allow for timely, well-planned treatment.

Just as the policies of the Bureau of Workers' Compensation frustrate injured workers, those of the U.S. Veterans Administration frustrate soldiers who sustained injuries in the war in Iran, the first Gulf War, or earlier conflicts. Many of these veterans have had to expend a great deal of time and energy fighting for appropriate treatment of health problems, such as chronic pain and disability.

Misunderstandings about the adequate treatment of chronic pain lie at the root of many of these failed policies. While systemic societal problems are not easily repaired, an essential first step toward improving social conditions will be the education of lawmakers and policymakers about the true nature of the chronic-pain experience. It is hoped this will achieve more visability in the proposed changes to health care in the United States.

Creating a National Pain Care Policy. Public support for better pain management has been building since October 2000, when former President Bill Clinton signed into law HR 3244, naming this the Decade of Pain Control and Research. This law acknowledged the place that pain and its control occupy in American health and cleared the way for funding pain-related research and treatment.

Notwithstanding the legislation, in 2004, the Drug Enforcement Agency withdrew its earlier endorsement of a set of prescribing guidelines for opioids, which had been crafted with the assistance of pain specialists. The American Academy of Pain Medicine and the American Pain Society continue to encourage a dialogue with regulators about the appropriate relationship between law and the practice of medicine.

"There are a lot of people trying to figure out how to engage [the DEA], but we're not able to get through the door," says Will Rowe of the American Pain Foundation. "Basically, the DEA has hung a 'do not disturb' sign outside its door and continues to scare doctors."

In recent years, the American Pain Foundation has shifted its advocacy efforts toward the House of Representatives, where Representative Mike Rogers, a Republican from Michigan, has repeatedly introduced the National Pain Care Policy Act. As of 2007 when this book was being prepared, Representative Lois Capps, a Democrat from California, had joined him in sponsoring bill HR 2994, with 35 cosponsors, in the House Subcommittee on Health during the 110th Congress. This was subsequently passed in the House, but awaits Senate confirmation.

Recognizing that advances in pain care to date have relied on trial-and-error discoveries, the bill calls for interdisciplinary research on the biology of pain, as well as a public information campaign to increase awareness of pain as a significant public health problem, an initiative to identify barriers to the delivery of appropriate pain care, and an outreach to underserved patient populations.

Like many of his cosponsors, Congressman Rogers has a personal interest in the passage of this bill. Rogers is a cancer

Voices of Pain

The American Pain Foundation website (*www.painfoundation. org*) includes profiles of patients who are coping with chronic pain. Its Voices of Pain feature allows you to hear these individuals describing their struggles with chronic pain as well as the stereotypes and discrimination that beset them from the public at large and even from the caregivers charged to serve them.

survivor, as is his father. In addition, he was moved by the plight of his brother Chuck, who underwent nearly 30 surgeries for chronic back pain. With young children and a wife to support, Chuck, a trained biologist, was unable to work because of his pain. Finally, Rogers located a pain clinic that helped Chuck to regain function.

After he first introduced the National Pain Care Policy Act, Representative Rogers's office was deluged with calls from pain support groups across the country. To continue the momentum, we encourage people in pain and their family members, physicians, and employers to contact their own U.S. representatives to voice their support. Describing how chronic pain affects an individual's life personalizes the problem of pain for policymakers, who will then be better able to understand its impact on the economy. Even more important is that the informed lawmaker might be persuaded to make greater policy efforts to improve the situation for the millions of Americans who live with chronic pain every day.

Chapter 10

The Future of Pain Management

P ain specialists are hopeful about the future. Our capacity to manage a broad range of pain syndromes is far greater today than we could imagine even ten years ago. This is largely due to the impressive gains made in research into pain pathways and mechanisms.

Laboratory research into the molecular and cellular components to pain are illuminating the basic mechanisms involved in chronic pain. Armed with this knowledge and the results of ongoing research with patients, we will develop ever more objective and accurate diagnostic tools. And as research uncovers genetic causes of pain and the effects of pain on the immune system, we will be able to provide more precisely targeted pain therapies.

In the future, research will translate into new drugs and new interventions. For example, suppose we could identify key proteins, or genetic markers, that would highlight the source of chronic pain in a given patient. Then imagine training a virus to target only those cells involved in the pain response. We might then be in a position to enfold a pain-blocking drug within the virus that would turn off the master switch for chronic pain in targeted cells. The patient's natural response to acute pain would remain undisturbed.

In our pursuit of pain control, brain-imaging studies also provide invaluable insights. We now know the locations of the brain that control pain, pain inhibition, and addiction. In addition, we are beginning to learn which parts of the brain correspond to the signaling of pain as opposed to suffering, for example, through the identification of the sites that control the emotions of anger and sadness.

Research such as this has already begun to pay dividends in the treatment and prevention of chronic pain.

Evolving Therapies

A brand-new class of non-narcotic analgesics, called N-type calcium channel blockers, has emerged to treat severe chronic pain. The first drug from this class, ziconotide (Prialt), is derived from a sea-snail venom. It is delivered through a surgically implanted catheter that delivers the drug into the fluid surrounding the spinal cord, where it blocks calcium channels that deliver pain signals to the brain.

Also encouraging, the use of pain pacemakers is expanding daily. Spinal cord stimulators are a well-established means of treating unremitting neuropathic pain. The low-level electrical current sent through the spinal cord reduces the intensity of pain signals, a process known as *neuromodulation.* We can also use neuromodulation to interfere with pain signals emanating from the peripheral nerves, closer to the site of pain.

One of the most exciting developments in pain therapy is the delivery of low-level electrical stimulation deep within the brain itself. *Deep brain stimulation* involves the implantation of a very fine electrode into the precise brain region that processes pain signals. The electrode delivers currents from a programmable transmitter implanted in the chest. This same approach has a track record of solid success in restoring function to patients with Parkinson's disease and other movement disorders, when medication has proven useless.

Will Doctors Be Able to Eliminate Chronic Pain Entirely?

Despite the exciting developments in research and pain therapy, there will never be a magic bullet, like a single drug, that will take care of all aspects that make up chronic pain. As new therapies emerge, their safety and effectiveness must be validated through evidence-based medicine. The use of promising but untested minimally invasive treatments can be tempting when the only alternative is major surgery. Though the literature about a new treatment may be compelling, only time and careful, comparative analyses will determine which treatments are most effective.

Of course, as new therapies are demonstrated to be effective, they will be absorbed into our ever-growing pain-management arsenal. But it's important to note that none of these strides in pain management will matter unless efforts at education and awareness accelerate.

Education on Two Fronts

As recently as 2005, the average pain patient saw 13 doctors before finding 1 who could help. In fact, pain specialists reported that 80 to 90 percent of their referrals came from patients, because other physicians didn't know that their specialty existed. Patients who are in pain benefit from timely treatment. It is clear that primary-care physicians are on the front line in deciding where to send patients with chronic pain—but often they don't know when, or where, to refer patients. Therefore, education is probably our most pressing need for the future of pain management. Efforts must be directed toward the community of health-care providers, the government, and the public.

Educating Physicians on the Web

To bridge the awareness gap, many pain specialists, including practitioners at the Cleveland Clinic, are working with state health departments to educate primary-care physicians about how to identify and treat chronic pain conditions in their patients. A Web-based training program and workshops are being developed in Germany to explain to family physicians the different types of chronic pain and how they are best treated. The first workshop delivered in the United States was held in Orlando, Florida, in February 2006. We hope that the family practitioners who participate in these programs will serve as ambassadors in their respective regions.

Also available for general practitioners who are interested in pain management is an interactive multimedia International Pain Course, on CD-ROM. To date, the CD-ROM has been translated into nine languages. In Germany alone, 28,000 general practitioners have been through the training it provides. The course was developed by an international advisory board supported by an unrestricted grant by Grunenthal, Aachen, Germany.

Establishing Pain Management as a Specialty

Currently, there are approximately 1,200 trained pain-management specialists in the United States. This falls far short of the number of pain-care professionals the country needs. Fortunately, with each passing year, more and more U.S. physicians are seeking out advanced training in pain management.

Traditionally, pain care was the province of anesthesiologists. More recently, psychologists have established practices devoted to pain management. Today, neurosurgeons, rehabilitation-medicine specialists, neurologists, and a handful of psychiatrists are seeking to specialize in pain management as well.

Pain Fellowships: A Start

Few universities and medical schools teach pain management as a specialty. Instead, physicians interested in pursuing pain care first earn board certification in their fields (for example, anesthesiology or neurology). They then must complete a 12- to 24-month fellowship in pain management.

Most of these fellowships are based in universities, but some are available in large private health-care institutions, such as the Cleveland Clinic, where they are overseen by the Accreditation Council for Graduate Medical Education (ACGME). Once admitted to the American Board of Medical Specialists (ABMS), a specialty such as pain medicine will be perceived in a different light by government agencies, like the U.S. Department of Veterans Affairs, the insurance industry, and other specialty organizations.

All pain-care fellows must meet training standards established by the ACGME. To determine if they meet those standards, they must sit for an examination at the end of their training. Passing the exam grants the physician a Certificate of Special Competence in Pain Management, which is awarded by the American Board of Anesthesiology. Two attempts to have pain management as a new medical discipline on the ABMS have been made. It will now only be a matter of time before its inclusion is accomplished.

As with painting a house—when you spend a month preparing surfaces before you actually begin to paint—the specialty of pain management is in the prepping phase now. Each small step we take builds the awareness, capacity, and resources required to meet our country's need for pain-care specialists. Ultimately, this will allow more patients to come to terms with their pain.

Mind Over Matter

We cannot cure chronic pain, but we can use our own psyches to divert attention from pain. Reynolds Price, an author and an English professor at Duke University, beautifully illustrates how this can be done in his book, *A Whole New Life: An Illness and a Healing.* In 1984, Price was diagnosed with cancer of the spinal cord. The pencil-thick tumor, ten inches long, ran "from my neck-hair downward," he wrote. After initial surgery failed to destroy the tumor, Price was stunned to learn that more surgery would result in death or quadriplegia.

To treat his cancer Price elected to undergo radiation therapy, which destroyed the nerves in his spine and paralyzed his legs. Price suffered a great deal of pain, and excessive doses of painkiller were prescribed by uncaring practitioners. Price slowly became dependent on morphine. With support from friends and the use of hypnosis, biofeedback, and antidepressants, Price slowly weaned himself from narcotics to the point where pain bothered him for no more than 15 minutes a day.

In the amazingly productive period since his recovery, Price has written 14 books.

"[I'm] not free from [pain's] constant presence in my body—it roars on still, round the clock every day, in my back and legs and across my shoulders—but [I'm] free from any real notice of it or concern for its presence, not to speak of the dread and the idiot regimen it forced upon me through three long years," he wrote.

But ask about his pain, and he cautions: "I'll quickly turn inward, watch the height of the blaze ... But it's you who've made me watch the fire and gauge it. Left alone with my body and mind, I'm not more focused on pain's existence than you'll be focused on the word *hippopotamus* at any moment unless I tell you not to think the word *hippopotamus* in the next 30 seconds."

For Price, the bonfire of pain is now in the background, largely because he has found something more worthwhile to do. "I write six days a week, long days that often run till bedtime; and the books are different from what came before in more ways than age. I sleep long nights with few hard dreams, and now I've outlived both my parents. Even my handwriting looks very little like the script of the man I was in June of '84. Cranky as it is, it's taller, more legible, with more air and stride. It comes down the arm of a grateful man."

Conclusion

People like Penney Cowan and Reynolds Price show us how meaningful life can be, even in the throes of chronic pain. If you take any message from this book, I hope it is that you can learn to live with pain—indeed, that you can live a very full and productive life. Most patients who suffer from pain wait anywhere from six months to several years before they seek help at a pain clinic. If you or a loved one develops chronic pain, please don't hesitate or wait to ask for help. All you have to do is seek trained professionals; modern medicine offers many pharmacological, interventional, and alternative therapies to ease your pain.

If you have endured symptoms of pain for three months or more, I offer the following suggestions:

- Do ask your family practitioner, internist, orthopedic surgeon, or other doctor to refer you to a pain specialist or a pain clinic.
- Don't expect to find a cure for your pain. The pain specialist will probably lay out the limitations of pain management on your first visit.

- Do expect the pain specialist to do his or her utmost to minimize your pain and improve your function; you will not be abandoned to suffer alone with your pain.

- Do tell the pain practitioner about all prior treatments you've undergone. Level with him or her about which treatments did not help and about any obstacles you encountered while seeking help.

- Do expect a number of treatment measures to be used concurrently to help you manage your pain. Pharmacological, interventional, and alternative therapies are rarely used in isolation.

- Don't be put off if you are referred to a psychologist or psychiatrist. Depression and pain go hand in hand, and many patients are unaware of the degree to which they are depressed. Behavioral therapy is not only recommended for individuals in chronic pain, it is a critical step of recovery.

- Do keep the faith. There is all the hope in the world that your ability to function will improve and that you will be able to make peace with your pain.

If you are close to someone with chronic pain:

- Do get involved. Become your loved one's advocate.

- Do conduct research on your own if the primary-care doctor cannot recommend any pain clinics or pain specialists.

- Don't be afraid to ask questions at the pain clinic. Be sure you understand what is being done and why certain combinations of pain blocks and drugs are necessary.

The appendixes of this book offer some resources to assist you or your loved one on the road to recovery.

Appendix 1

Suggested Resources

The organizations below can serve as starting points on the quest for further information about chronic pain.

American Alliance of Cancer Pain Initiatives
c/o School of Medicine & Public Health,
1300 University Avenue, Room 4720
Madison, Wisconsin 53706
(608) 265-4013
Email: *aacpi@mailplus.wisc.edu*
www.aacpi.wisc.edu

American Chronic Pain Association
Box 850
Rocklin, California 95677-0850
(916) 632-0922 or 800-533-3231
Email: *acpa@pacbell.net*
www.theacpa.org

American Council for Headache Education
19 Mantua Road
Mt. Royal, New Jersey 08061
(856) 423-0258 or 800-255-2243
Email: *achehq@talley.com*
www.achenet.org

American Fibromyalgia Syndrome Association
6380 E. TanqueVerde, Suite D
Tucson, Arizona 85715
(520) 733-1570
www.afsafund.org

American Pain Foundation
201 North Charles Street, Suite 710
Baltimore, Maryland 21201-4111
888-615-7246
Email: *info@painfoundation.org*
www.painfoundation.org

Arthritis Foundation
1330 West Peachtree Street, Suite 100
Atlanta, Georgia 30309
(404) 872-7100, (404) 965-7888, or 800-568-4045
Email: *help@arthritis.org*
www.arthritis.org

Mayday Fund for Pain Research
c/o SPG
136 West 21st Street, 6th Floor
New York, New York 10011
(212) 366-6970
Email: *mayday@maydayfund.org*
www.painandhealth.org

Myositis Association of America
1233 20th Street NW, Suite 402
Washington, D.C. 20036
(202) 887-0088
Email: *tma@myositis.org*
www.myositis.org

National Chronic Pain Outreach Association
Box 274
Millboro, Virginia 24460
(540) 862-9437
www.chronicpain.org

National Chronic Pain Society
8711 Town Park Drive, # 2116
Houston, Texas 77036
(281) 357-4673
Email: *ncps@houston.rr.com*
www.ncps-cpr.org

National Foundation for the Treatment of Pain
Box 70045
Houston, Texas 77270
(713) 862-9332
Email: *jfshmd@houston.rr.com*
www.paincare.org

National Headache Foundation
820 N. Orleans, Suite 217
Chicago, Illinois 60610-3132
(773) 388-6399 or 888-643-5552
Email: *info@headaches.org*
www.headaches.org

National Institute of Dental and Craniofacial Research
National Institutes of Health, DHHS
45 Center Drive, Rm. 4AS19 MSC 6400
Bethesda, Maryland 20892-6400
(301) 496-4261
Email: *nidrinfo@od31.nidr.nih.gov*
www.nidr.nih.gov

National Pain Foundation
300 E. Hampden Ave., Suite 100
Englewood, Colorado 80113
(866) 590-7246
Email: *npf@nationalpainfoundation.org*
www.NationalPainFoundation.org

Partners Against Pain
1 Stamford Forum
Stamford, Connecticut 06901-3431
888-726-7535 (option #5)
Email: *partnersagainstpain@pharma.com*
www.partnersagainstpain.com

Reflex Sympathetic Dystrophy Syndrome Association
Box 502
Milford, Connecticut 06460
(203) 877-3790 or 877-662-7737 (toll-free)
Email: *info@rsds.org*
www.rsds.org

Trigeminal Neuralgia Association
925 Northwest 56th Terrace, Suite C
Gainesville, Florida 32605-6402
800-923-3608
Email: *tnanational@tna-support.org*
www.tna-support.org

Appendix 2

Measuring Pain

Quantifying how much pain a patient is feeling is crucial to its treatment. Several psychological tools define the overall pain experience expressed by a patient. The Visual Analog Score (VAS) and its variations are simple numbered systems that reveal the level of pain at a given moment.

To evaluate the overall impact of chronic pain, various pain assessment questionnaires were developed. The McGill Pain Assessment Questionnaire (MPQ), developed by Ronald Melzack, takes an inventory of a patient's symptoms. It has four parts:

Pain Assessment Questionnaire

(adapted from the MPQ)

Part 1: Patient data

On the following body diagram, mark the location of your pain, and mark areas where you feel the pain using indicators E for external, I for internal, or both.

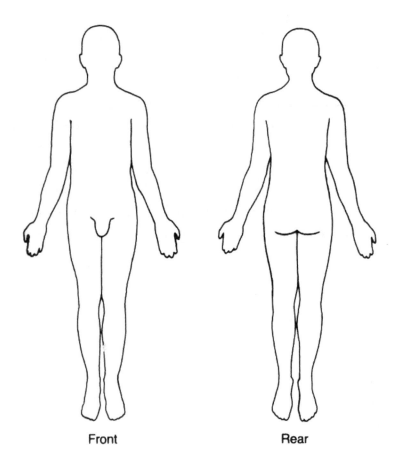

Front   Rear

Part 2: What does your pain feel like?

Some of the words below describe your present pain. Circle *only* those words that best describe it. Leave out any category that is not suitable. Use only a single word in each appropriate category—the one that applies best.

Sensory 1–8	Affective 9–15	Evaluative 16	Miscellaneous 17–20
1 Flickering Quivering Pulsing Throbbing Beating Pounding	**2** Jumping Flashing Shooting	**3** Pricking Boring Drilling Stabbing Lancinating	**4** Sharp Cutting Lacerating
5 Pinching Pressing Gnawing Cramping Crushing	**6** Tugging Pulling Wrenching	**7** Hot Burning Scalding Searing	**8** Tingling Itchy Smarting Stinging
9 Dull Sore Hurting Aching Heavy	**10** Tender Taut Rasping Splitting	**11** Tiring Exhausting	**12** Sickening Suffocating
13 Fearful Frightful Terrifying	**14** Punishing Grueling Cruel Vicious Killing	**15** Wretched Blinding	**16** Annoying Troublesome Miserable Intense Unbearable
17 Spreading Radiating Penetrating Piercing	**18** Tight Numb Drawing Squeezing Tearing	**19** Cool Cold Freezing	**20** Nagging Nauseating Agonizing Dreadful Torturing

Part 3: How does your pain change over time?

A) Which word or words would you use to describe the pattern of your pain?
   1. Continuous, Steady, Constant
   2. Rhythmic, Periodic, Intermittent
   3. Brief, Momentary, Transient

B) What relieves your pain?

C) What increases your pain?

Part 4: How strong is your pain?

People agree that the following five words represent pain of increasing intensity. They are:

1	2	3	4	5
Mild	Discomforting	Distressing	Horrible	Excruciating

To answer each question below, write the number of the most appropriate word in the space beside the question.

1) Which word describes your pain right now?   _____

2) Which word describes your pain at its worst?   _____

3) Which word describes your pain when at its least?   _____

4) Which word describes the worst toothache   _____
   you've ever had?

5) Which word describes the worst headache   _____
   you've ever had?

6) Which word describes the worst stomachache   _____
   you've ever had?

Other Pain Questionnaires

Another questionnaire administered to people with chronic pain is the Beck Depression Inventory, or BDI. This psychological instrument assesses a patient's level of depression. It consists of 21 questions; individuals are asked to rank the severity of each item and to choose the statement that best suits their own perception. The advantage of the BDI is that it has been used extensively for 30 years. It takes only ten minutes to administer and score.

The Minnesota Multiphasic Personality Inventory (MMPI-2), a second evaluation commonly used by psychologists, measures overall psychological status and is considered the gold standard in assessment. It is comprehensive and available in long and short forms.

These psychological instruments are used to aid the course of multidisciplinary pain management. When added to the activity diary the patient is asked to keep for two weeks, this background information gives the health-care provider insight into the impact of pain on daily functioning. An activity diary should include:

- Amount of time spent sitting, standing, walking, or reclining
- Which medications are taken, and of what type
- Pain level
- Time of day for each notation

Sample Pain Diary

Name: _____

	Describe situation ⬇	Sensation (1–10) ⬇	Describe sensation ⬇

Monday, November 1

Time 1	8 A.M.	Breakfast	6	Achy
Time 2	Noon	Lunch	8	Throbbing
Time 3	9 P.M.	Bedtime	10	Sharp
		Total:	24	
		Average:	8	

Tuesday, November 2

Time 1	8:30 A.M.	Breakfast	9	Sharp spasms
Time 2	11:30 A.M.	Getting up	7	Throbbing
Time 3	9 P.M.	Paying bills	5	Sore
		Total:	21	
		Average:	7	

Wednesday, November 3

Time 1	8 A.M.	Getting up	4	Sore
Time 2	Noon	Lunch	5	Sore
Time 3	10 P.M.	Dinner out	6	Achy
		Total:	15	
		Average:	5	

Distress (1–10)	Describe distress	Action taken or medications
5	Frustrated	Shower
8	Disgusted	2 ibuprofin
10	Helpless	Heating pad
Total: 23		
Average: 8		

Distress (1–10)	Describe distress	Action taken or medications
10	Scared	Go back to bed
8	Sad	RR, heat
4	Comforted	Paced activities
Total: 22		
Average: 7		

Distress (1–10)	Describe distress	Action taken or medications
2	Relief	Gentle exercise
1	In control	RR, 2 aspirin
1	Happy	Hot shower on return
Total: 4		
Average: 1		

Appendix 3

Analgesics: A Quick Reference

*A*nalgesics are medicines used to relieve pain. Doctors may prescribe two types. *Opioid analgesics* are narcotics, derived from opium. *Nonopioid analgesics* are not considered narcotics.

Common Opioids

- Morphine
- Morphine—Controlled Release (MS-Contin, Oramorph SR)
- Morphine—Controlled Release (Kadian)
- Hydromorphone hydrochloride (Dilaudid)
- Meperidine (Demerol)
- Fentanyl (Sublimaze, Duragesic)
- Codeine (Tylenol with Codeine #2, #3, or #4)
- Acetaminophen and hydrocodone (Vicodin, Lortab)

- Oxycodone and acetaminophen (Percodan, Percocet, Tylox, Roxicet, Roxicodone)
- Oxycodone Controlled Release (OxyContin)
- Methadone (Dolophine)
- Propoxyphene napsylate and acetaminophen (Darvon, Darvocet)

The use of opioids may produce drug side effects, which may become more common as doses are increased, for example, in the treatment of severe pain. Side effects include nausea and vomiting, constipation, pruritis (itching), mental confusion, sedation, respiratory depression, and hypersensitivity (allergic) reactions. Proper use of opioids in patients with severe pain includes managing these side effects rather than discontinuing the drug's use.

Common Nonopioids

- Tramadol (Ultram)
- Ketorolac tromethamine (Toradol)
- Ibuprofen (Motrin, Advil)
- Acetaminophen (Tylenol)
- Aspirin
- Naproxen sodium (Aleve, Naprosyn)

Appendix 4

*Simple Exercises
for the Hands and Arms*

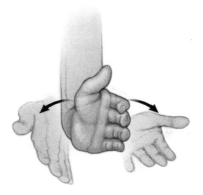

Wrist exercises: Pronation, supination

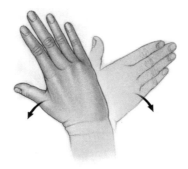

Lateral movement at the wrist, with fingers extended

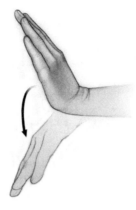

Flexion-extension exercises at the wrist, with fingers extended

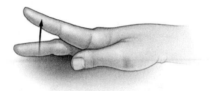

With the hand flat on the table, each finger is individually raised (extended), to greatest degree possible

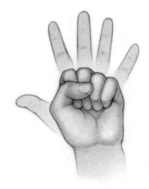

Making a fist, with extension of fingers (a continuation of flexion-extension exercise)

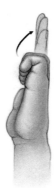

Flexion and extension of the fingers, at the palm

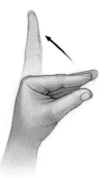

Pincer movement of all fingers against extended thumb

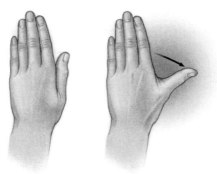

Maximum thumb-extension exercises

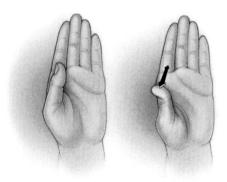

Thumb-to-index finger exercises

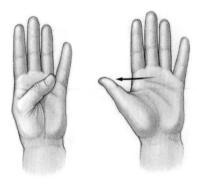

Thumb exercises, as shown

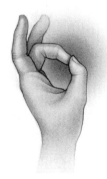

Individual finger-thumb movements

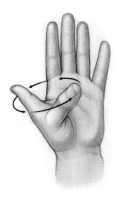

Rotation of thumb, as shown

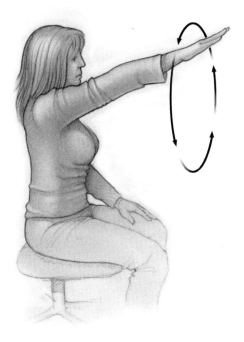

Shoulder rotation with arm outstretched

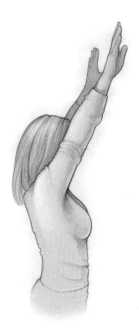

Extension of shoulders, with arms outstretched

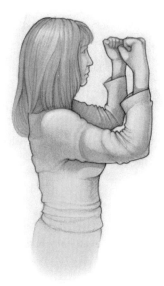

Flexion at elbows, with hands in a fist

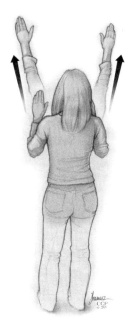

Extension exercise for shoulder and arm

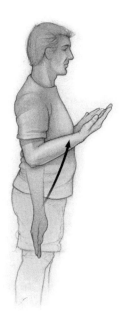

Extension exercises, at elbow

Index

About the Author

Michael Stanton-Hicks, MD, is vice chairman of the Anesthesiology Institute at Cleveland Clinic in Cleveland, Ohio. His clinical interests are chronic pain, complex regional pain syndrome, and regional anesthesia. Dr. Stanton-Hicks is board-certified in both pain medicine and anesthesiology.

A frequent national and international lecturer, Dr. Stanton-Hicks has authored more than 150 articles, book chapters, and textbooks. He is an active member of numerous national and international professional societies, having been president and committee chairman of many of these organizations. Dr. Stanton-Hicks has received several distinguished awards for his activities in pain medicine and continues to be principal investigator for numerous funded research projects.

About Cleveland Clinic

Cleveland Clinic, located in Cleveland, Ohio, is a not-for-profit multispecialty academic medical center that integrates clinical and hospital care with research and education.

Cleveland Clinic was founded in 1921 by four renowned physicians with a vision of providing outstanding patient care based upon the principles of cooperation, compassion, and innovation. *U.S. News & World Report* consistently names Cleveland Clinic as one of the nation's best hospitals in its annual "America's Best Hospitals" survey. Approximately 1,800 full-time salaried physicians and researchers at Cleveland Clinic and Cleveland Clinic Florida represent more than 100 medical specialties and subspecialties. In 2007 there were 3.5 million outpatient visits to Cleveland Clinic and 50,455 hospital admissions. Patients came for treatment from every state and from more than 80 countries. Cleveland Clinic's website address is *www.clevelandclinic.org.*